WOMEN'S
SEXUAL
HEALTH

WOMEN'S
SEXUAL
HEALTH

RUTH STEINBERG, M.D.
and
LINDA ROBINSON, R.N., C.N.M.

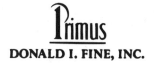

DONALD I. FINE, INC.

New York

To our mothers
L. J. R.
R. S.

CONTENTS

WOMEN'S
SEXUAL
HEALTH

$\mathscr{I}$NTRODUCTION

$\mathscr{S}$ex, like food, can and should be extraordinarily pleasurable. Given the right menu and carefully chosen company, both can be activities that afford passion and joy. Excess in either pursuit can lead to diminution of self-image, destruction of self-respect, disease, and death. But a woman who can look in the mirror and feel proud of herself can savor life's sensual pleasures.

Historically, women have been discouraged from being proud of their bodies. The "ideal woman" as represented by the fashion and advertising industries is extraordinarily tall, painfully thin, and hairless. Women's fashions dictate that women shave their body hair and mask their body odor. When they compare themselves to what is "fashionable," most women are led to believe that their bodies don't measure up. Their breasts are too large, too small, too far apart, too droopy, or too pointy. Yet women must become comfortable with themselves in order to enjoy good mental, physical, and sexual health. The "sexy woman" is not that anorexic, hairless giant, but the woman who understands and enjoys her body and is proud of it. Self-esteem is sexy.

Knowing how your body works is empowering. It allows you to understand your body's limitations and to fully utilize its capabilities. Sexual education should be part of overall health education, incorporated into our teaching programs early on so that young girls can learn to be proud of themselves. Sexual awareness does not lead to promiscuity, but it can lead to increased self-esteem, awareness of choices in sexuality, and responsible decision making.

Knowing who you are and how your body works is the basis for making informed sexual choices. Although men and women share the pleasure of sex and the risk of sexually transmitted diseases (STDs), it is the women who must bear the reproductive consequences.

Many diseases besides acquired immune deficiency syndrome (AIDS) have disastrous effects for women if left undiagnosed and untreated. Many of these diseases can lead to infertility or predispose women to cancer. You should know the risk factors, symptoms, and treatments for these diseases and have health-care providers who will give the information and support you need to make informed choices.

1

$\mathcal{T}$HE
BASIC FACTS

$\mathcal{M}$any of us reach puberty and begin to menstruate without much information from our mothers on how our bodies work. Much of our information (or misinformation) is picked up from friends or from books. When problems arise, women begin to ask questions.

There is a good reason why our mothers never explained the reproductive system to us: Many of them never understood it themselves, and many were too embarrassed to talk about it. A woman's reproductive system is actually a very complex balance of structures and hormones. The basic explanation that "Daddy has the seed and Mommy has the egg, and if the two don't meet, you bleed" will get you through life, but really understanding your body and how it works is an important aspect of womanhood. A prepubescent girl of age nine will most likely not understand an in-depth lecture on reproductive endocrinology, but an honest education should start early.

In our culture, the onset of menstruation (menarche) has traditionally been looked upon and portrayed as a negative event. It differs from every other developmental milestone in this way. We are ecstatic at our child's first word, applaud her first step, celebrate joyously when she is toilet trained, and happily play the tooth fairy at the loss of her baby teeth. But when a girl begins to menstruate, the sentiment is more often, "Well, too bad the carefree days are over." Menstruation is nicknamed "my friend" or "the curse," which implies that we can't even speak its name.

Making babies is not just magic. It is a fascinating system that enables almost every woman to create life. Menstruation is not a shameful curse to dread each month, and should never be so explained to a young girl expecting her first menses, or menstrual flow. With menstruation comes the power to create life, which makes the menstrual flow something to celebrate. It also carries with it a responsibility that should be addressed. No girl should ever begin to menstruate without knowing why and what is happening, and how babies are conceived.

THE FEMALE ANATOMY

There are many structures that constitute the female reproductive system. Each has its own function and is crucial to the whole system. It's difficult for very young girls to clearly differentiate their external reproductive organs. Boys can see and handle their penises, so it's easier for them to visualize how their reproductive systems work. Not only are girls' sexual organs more concealed, but girls are also often discouraged from touching them, and many girls develop a sense that their reproductive organs are mysterious and somehow forbidden.

External Organs

Breasts.   Breasts are mammary glands, a distinguishing feature of female mammals. These glands are used for feeding our young for the first year or two of life. In humans, the breasts are made up of milk glands and fat and can vary greatly in size. However, the size of a woman's breasts in no way determines how capable she is of nursing her babies. Very small breasts are quite capable of producing adequate amounts of milk. The breasts begin to develop at puberty. First the nipples enlarge and then the mass of the breast follows. This coincides with the initial growth of body hair, especially in the pubic area and in the armpits.

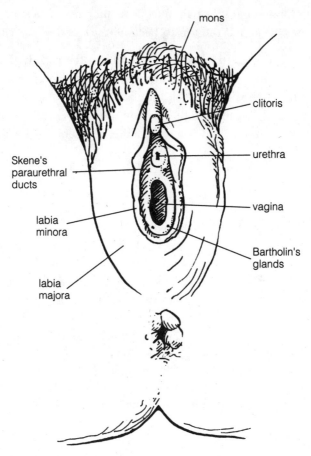

Figure 1.1. External Organs

Vulva. The vulva is the area that includes the external genital organs. The labia (lips) consist of two large folds of skin that cover and protect the female genitals. The labia majora (large lips) are covered with hair after puberty and are the most external of the two pairs. The labia majora connect with the soft, fatty, hair-covered area over the pubic bone called the mons. The labia minora (small lips) are mucous membranes, not skin, and are therefore not covered with hair. They are pink in color and moist like all mucous membranes. The labia minora are narrow and join at the top to become the hood of the clitoris.

Clitoris. At the junction of the labial folds is the clitoris. This is an erectile organ that becomes firm with sexual stimulation. The clitoris is the center of female sexual pleasure and is embryologically equivalent to the male's penis. Both are composed of erectile tissue, and when the human fetus is developing, either the penis or the clitoris is derived from the same structural bud.

Internal Organs

Cervix. The cervix is the necklike opening to the uterus. It is a smooth, firm structure composed of elastic and connective tissue with some muscle fibers that protrude into the vagina. In nonpregnant women, the cervix is pink in color, and the opening is closed and firm. It looks like a tiny doughnut with the hole closed. During pregnancy, the cervix becomes engorged with blood, and it will soften and turn purplish in color. The cervix is the organ that dilates during childbirth to allow the passage of the baby from the uterus into the birth canal.

Fallopian tubes. At the top of the uterus are two tubes, one going out from either side. These tubes are the passageways through which the eggs pass from the ovaries into the uterus. They are also a route for the sperm to travel to meet the egg, and the sperm fertilizes the egg in the fallopian tube. These tubes are lined with specialized cells that secrete enzymes to nourish and propel the egg along its route to the uterus.

Ovaries.   At the end of each fallopian tube is an oval-shaped organ that produces and houses ova, or eggs. Each ovary produces one egg every other month, so the ovaries generally alternate to produce one egg each month. (If surgical removal of one ovary is ever necessary, the other ovary will compensate for this loss.) The process of producing an egg is called ovulation. The ovaries also produce many hormones, including estrogen and progesterone, that are essential in the reproductive process.

In humans, the female has already developed a maximum number of eggs (6 million to 7 million) by the time she is a 20-week-old fetus in her mother's womb. At birth a newborn female has 1 million to 2 million eggs. Once a young woman reaches puberty, she has approximately 300,000 to 400,000 eggs remaining. A hormonal switch is then turned on so that the eggs mature in a programmed manner until the woman reaches menopause (cessation of menstruation). Since all of a woman's eggs are present from birth, their exposure to environmental hazards is cumulative over the woman's lifetime. In contrast, the life cycle of sperm is only 90 days. Long-term exposure to environmental hazards, therefore, affect eggs much more than they do sperm.

Uterus.   The uterus, also known as the womb, is the organ that nourishes and protects a growing fetus until birth. In nonpregnant women, the uterus is about the size of a small pear, and similarly shaped. It is firm and elastic, consisting of three layers: The inner lining is called the endometrium, whose top part is shed during menstruation. The middle layer, called the myometrium, is a thick, smooth muscle. The thin outer layer is called the perimetrium.

Vagina.   The vagina is an expandable pocket of tissue surrounded by layers of muscle. It is the organ that receives the male penis during intercourse and is the receptacle for the ejaculated sperm. During orgasm the vagina contracts spasmodically, thereby helping the sperm to move up into the uterus to meet the egg. (However, pregnancy can occur without a female orgasm.) The top of the vagina forms the sidewalls of the cervix (the mouth of the uterus). During childbirth,

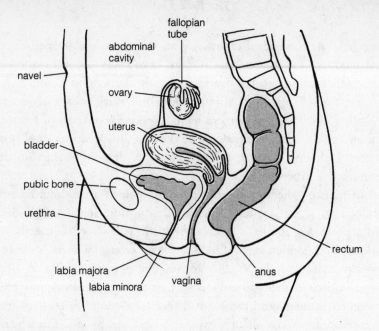

Figure 1.2. Internal Organs

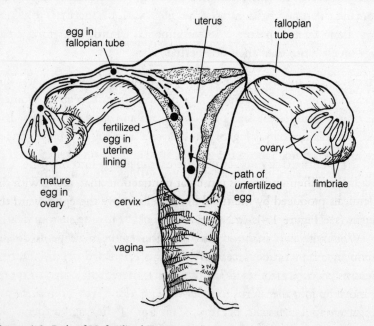

Figure 1.3. Path of Unfertilized Egg

the baby passes through the uterus and the vagina becomes the birth canal.

REVIEW OF THE MONTHLY,
OR MENSTRUAL, CYCLE

The monthly cycle, also called the menstrual cycle, is an intricate part of the female reproductive system. It is a continuous process with different phases that gradually progress from one to the next in a natural flow. These phases are constantly preparing a woman for pregnancy.

The reproductive cycle actually starts in a portion of the brain called the hypothalamus, where the very complex balance of hormones begins. The hypothalamus produces and releases substances called releasing factors, which travel down a connecting stalk to the anterior pituitary gland. The releasing factors are so named because they stimulate the anterior pituitary to release several hormones, two of which stimulate the ovaries. Those hormones are called follicle-stimulating hormone (FSH) and luteinizing hormone (LH).

The FSH and LH produce changes in the ovaries that stimulate maturation of an egg. At ovulation, the surface of the ovary actually ruptures and an egg is released into the fallopian tube. At the entrance of the fallopian tubes are fimbriae—fingerlike structures that move to and fro over the ovary and sweep the extruded egg into the tube. The tubular wall then undergoes muscular contractions that, along with the chemicals produced by the tubal lining cells, move the egg toward the uterus (see Figure 1.4).

When the egg is introduced into the fallopian tube, the ovary produces an increased amount of progesterone, the hormone that prepares the uterine lining to nourish a fertilized egg. If at this time sexual intercourse results in the fertilization of the egg, the level of progesterone increases even more. If the egg is not fertilized, the progesterone level will eventually drop, about 10 to 12 days after ovula-

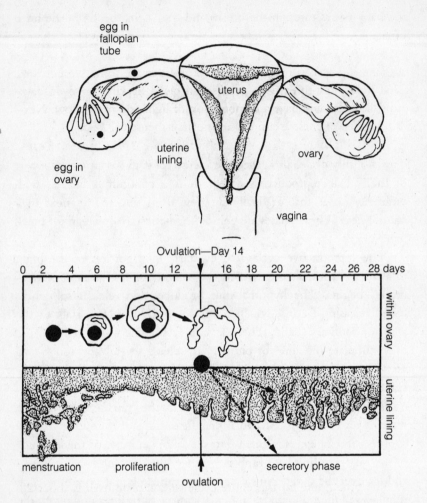

Figure 1.4. Menstrual Cycle

tion. This decrease in the progesterone level causes menstrual bleeding, which begins exactly 14 days after the egg is released.

The Menstrual Cycle

The menstrual cycle consists of three phases. The first is the menstrual phase, during which menstrual bleeding occurs. The first day of bleeding is counted as day one of the menstrual cycle. During this initial phase, the lining of the uterus is sloughed off and then discarded through the cervix and the vagina, and leaves the body. This process can take a few days or even longer. For example, some women will bleed lightly for three days, others will bleed heavily for seven days, and still others will have a combination of light and heavy flow. Nevertheless, all of these examples are normal menstrual periods.

After the menstrual phase, the proliferative phase begins. At this point there is an increased production of estrogen due to FSH release by the pituitary gland. Estrogen stimulates the uterine lining to repair itself and causes the ovary to start the maturation process of the egg.

The secretory phase (also called the luteal phase) follows ovulation. LH released from the pituitary causes progesterone to be secreted in increased amounts. This causes a further buildup of the endometrium in anticipation of fertilization and implantation of an egg. At the time of ovulation, vaginal secretions become noticeably thinner and more copious in order to facilitate the fertilization process. Also during this phase, the penis can enter the vagina more easily, and with less stimulation. The ejaculated sperm can enter the cervix more easily because the mucus is thinner and allows for better motility. This phase is also the time when your sex drive (libido) is most likely to increase. Because of all these factors, it is the time when fertilization is most likely to occur. If fertilization does not occur, there is a decrease in hormone production at the end of the secretory phase, which causes the uterine lining to shrink and the menstrual blood flow to eventually start again.

The time frame for this entire cycle to complete itself is about 28 days. These days are counted from the beginning of one menstrual period to the beginning of the next (day one of bleeding to the next day one of bleeding). The number of days that you bleed has nothing to do with the length of the cycle. Women who bleed for three days and women who bleed for eight days may both still have a 28-day cycle. Although 28 days is the average length of a menstrual cycle, the cycle may vary a bit from woman to woman and from cycle to cycle in the same woman. About 90 percent of women have menstrual cycles of 23 to 35 days. The way to determine the length of your own cycle is to consistently record the first day of bleeding and count from there. Doing this for six cycles will give you a good idea of your pattern.

Young girls who are just starting to menstruate may have very irregular cycles, and that is normal. There may be three or four months between periods, or only three weeks. Sometimes it can take up to five years before the cycle regulates itself into a recognizable pattern. Medically this is not a problem, but socially it may be extremely disruptive to the lifestyle of a young teenager. The important point to remember is that once a girl has begun to menstruate, she is capable of becoming pregnant. Ovulation and periods may be very irregular, but conception can take place. With very irregular cycles it is extremely difficult to know when a young girl is most fertile, so she should consider herself always fertile. Making the decision to become sexually active and taking responsibility for it are discussed in the next chapter.

Discharge. The vagina is not a sterile environment: It is filled with bacteria that are normal vaginal inhabitants and that make up its natural cleansing system. There is always some type of mucous vaginal fluid present. Therefore, when something is introduced into the vagina (semen, for example), the vagina will cleanse itself by the natural downward and outward flow of these fluids. The vaginal discharge you notice between menstrual periods needs no special attention. During normal bathing or showers, clean the outside areas of the vagina with mild soap. Douching (cleaning the vagina with a water solution introduced by an applicator) is not necessary. Perfumed douches should not be used. The introduction of a perfumed substance into the vagina may make it more susceptible to infection and irritation, or may cause allergic reactions. The normal vaginal discharge has a mild, musty odor, which is not offensive or even noticeable. Cosmetic companies, however, have promoted the idea that the normal state of a woman's genitals is unclean or unappealing. TV ads bombard women with products to mask their natural body odors. These nostrums are not necessary and may even be harmful, causing allergic reactions and irritation.

Pads and tampons. During menstruation some type of product is needed to absorb the flow of menstrual blood. There are a multitude of products to choose from in the form of pads or tampons. In the last decade, a great improvement has been made in the design of sanitary pads. The old belts with metal clasps and large bulky pads are now passé. Pads with adhesive backing and a natural contour are much more comfortable. Some of the newer pads, however, have added perfume. These chemicals are not needed and, as with perfumed douches, may cause local irritation in some women. The menstrual flow does have its own distinct odor—a musty smell slightly stronger than that of ordinary vaginal discharge. However, the only time this odor is noticeable is when you are changing your pad. Passersby certainly cannot detect the odor of a woman's menstrual period. Therefore, there is no need for perfumes; they serve no purpose whatsoever.

Tampons offer much more freedom of movement during the menstrual period than do pads, and they are a safe and reliable alternative. Young girls may initially have difficulty using tampons if the hymen is still intact. The hymen is a thin membrane that tightly rings the vaginal opening in young girls. It was once thought that the hymen stayed intact until the first act of sexual penetration, but this is not usually the case. In fact, the tissue may be broken by strenuous activity or by masturbation. For this reason, no young girl should be dissuaded from using tampons. If a girl is able to use tampons, it does not mean she was or is sexually active. Women who are sexually active may even experience a few days of vaginal dryness following tampon use, because the tampons absorb not only the menstrual blood but also the vaginal secretions. It may take a day or two for the vagina to replenish itself. Therefore, the use of a water-based lubricant such as K-Y jelly may make intercourse more comfortable. During and immediately after one's period, the vagina cleanses itself. Again, there is no need to douche.

Menstrual Symptoms

There are varying symptoms that women may experience throughout the menstrual cycle. Some are pleasurable, like increased libido and energy, but some are uncomfortable, especially if they are not properly understood.

Cramps.   Cramps, or lower abdominal pains, are a common symptom of the menstrual cycle. Cramps are likely to occur as the uterine lining breaks down and begins to be passed through the cervix. Spasms can occur as the larger clots get forced through a very small opening. Cramps may also be caused by the effects of progesterone, which slows down the gastrointestinal system. During the secretory phase there is a chance that cramps might be caused by a sluggish bowel. Cramps are more common in women who have not borne children, but they may be experienced by all women. They may recur or increase in premenopausal women. Once a woman has had a child, however, the opening of the cervix is a little bit bigger and softer and, therefore, not as likely to go into spasm.

Cramps themselves are not an indication of a serious problem. Many women just live with them, since they are temporary. The pain from the cramps, though, may be intense enough to interfere with a woman's normal activities. If this is the case, and it continues from one cycle to the next, there are a few relief measures to be employed. It's always better to start with simple remedies and go from there.

For cramps that occur the day before your period or the first two days of your period, one very effective treatment is heat. Applying heat on the lower abdomen will relax the muscles and make the spasms less intense. A warm bath is probably most effective, as that will relax your whole body. If this is impractical, applying heat on just the abdomen will help. A hot-water bottle or heating pad may be very comforting. A hot-water bottle is a very useful device because you don't need to be near an electrical outlet to use one. The one drawback is that a bottle is heavier than a heating pad, and that may add to your abdominal discomfort. A hot-water bottle should not be excessively hot and should be wrapped in a towel to avoid skin burns. A heating pad should not be left on a high setting, as this may also cause skin burns, especially if you fall asleep with it on. Try them both to see which you prefer. Warm drinks, such as herbal teas, may also relieve abdominal cramps. Herbalists suggest that peppermint tea may be particularly effective.

If this treatment is not practical, the next step is a mild pain reliever. Ibuprofen is very effective in the relief of menstrual cramps. This is not a harmful drug, and it is readily available over the counter. It inhibits the release of prostaglandins, which are substances released by the uterus during menses and which induce cramping. If this medication, taken every four to six hours, does not sufficiently relieve your cramps to the point where you can function normally, you should call your health-care provider for a checkup. There may be some underlying problem that is causing such severe symptoms.

It was once thought that reducing salt intake during a woman's period would reduce her cramps. This has not been borne out in scientific studies, and unless you have severe kidney impairment, your salt intake need not be restricted.

Premenstrual syndrome (PMS).   Premenstrual syndrome, commonly known as PMS, has become a sort of catchall term for a variety of symptoms and complaints. There is a specific clinical definition of PMS that is used in diagnosing the condition. First of all, the symptoms of PMS (and they can vary widely) must occur cyclically. Second, the symptoms occur during the secretory phase (luteal phase) which begins after ovulation and ends with the menstrual flow. This is followed by a symptom-free period of at least one week. Finally, the symptoms must be severe enough to interfere with work, home life, or interpersonal relationships.

In recent years there have been many studies devoted to PMS, but still the actual cause is unknown. There are many theories, but none has been proved scientifically. The emotional symptoms of PMS include anger, hostility, intolerance of others, emotional instability, anxiety, and depression. In addition, many women experience physical symptoms, including fatigue, headache, constipation, joint pain, abdominal bloating, breast tenderness, and acne. PMS does not seem to be related to a woman's age, since menstruating women of all ages experience it. However, women in their thirties seem to seek treatment for PMS more often. Unfortunately, there is no one surefire treatment for the condition.

If you are suffering symptoms of PMS, there are several things you can do before you go to your health-care provider. The first step is to make monthly charts of your symptoms so the pattern can be established (see Figure 1.4, page 10). Day one of the chart is the first day of your period and should be marked as such. Fill in the remarkable symptoms you had on that day (i.e., cramps, bloating, heavy flow, headache, irritability). Also fill in what you ate and what you did for exercise on that day. This is time-consuming at first, but it is very important to complete a chart every day for a full three cycles. It's the only way to see exactly what your pattern is, and it will give you and your health-care provider a much better idea of how to treat the symptoms.

PMS can often be treated with modifications in your diet or with regular exercise, which releases endorphins, naturally occurring substances that relieve pain and may elevate mood. It is always better to start with simple changes like these and evaluate their effectiveness before going on to medication or something invasive. Some treatments include vitamin B_6 (not exceeding 200 mg/day), vitamin E (400 mg/day), ibuprofen (600 mg every six hours until bleeding starts), or birth control pills. The treatment of PMS is hit-or-miss at best. There are many medical theories for the causes of PMS. None of these theories have been successfully substantiated. There are as many treatments as there are theories. What works well for one person may not work at all for another. You should discuss treatment options with your health care provider.

Pain during ovulation.   Some women are very aware of the time of ovulation because they feel some pain in the lower abdomen (this is called *mittelschmerz,* or "middle pain"). The pain is thought to be caused by the discharge of fluid from around the egg as it is released. The discomfort may vary from a dull ache to a sharp stabbing pain, depending on the cycle and on the individual woman. This pain should not last more than three days and usually responds well to ibuprofen. There may also be a small amount of spotting (bleeding) associated with ovulation, but this is not worrisome. Such symptoms do not require an office visit.

2

$\mathcal{M}$AKING DECISIONS ABOUT SEX

$\mathcal{F}$rom puberty until menopause, women's bodies are continually preparing for reproduction. With the availability of birth control methods, we can make conscious decisions about whether or not we want to reproduce at all, and if so, when.

Throughout nature, sex is performed for reproductive purposes. For human beings, though, having sex is far more complex than it is for other animals. There is enormous conflict between our animal instincts telling us to do it and our social conscience saying "Wait until you're married," "I don't know him (or her) well enough," "He (or she) might have some disease," or "I might get pregnant."

Societal constraints have been very powerful forces, but not powerful enough to keep women from having sex. Our instincts prove to be much stronger than any social rules. What has resulted is plenty of guilt, sexually transmitted diseases (STDs), and unwanted pregnancy, because in the past women would rather deny that they wanted sex than be adequately prepared for it. Although women's sexual needs may differ from men's, women want and enjoy sex. They also bear the responsibility and consequences for it: Women get pregnant, but men do not.

Both men and women get sexually transmitted diseases, but women are more often scarred for life from them.

There are several reliable birth control measures available to almost everyone. And sexually transmitted diseases are preventable. All decisions about having sex should be informed ones based on the risks, pleasures, and insights into oneself. This decision-making process shifts and changes as women age.

The key to satisfying sex at any age is deciding that this is what you want. Second, open communication between you and your partner will make sex a much more satisfying experience. And taking and sharing responsibility for protecting yourself from an unwanted pregnancy or STD's allows you to let go of anxiety and focus on this very pleasurable, exciting experience.

SEXUAL CHOICES

Sexual choices, such as the number of partners (at one time or in a lifetime), the sex of the partner, or the frequency of sex, are made in response to biological and psychosocial needs. The urge for sexual release can sometimes lead to unfortunate and unplanned results. Don't make sexual decisions if drugs or alcohol have clouded your judgment. Learn your own body's sexual needs, and if you are comfortable satisfying those needs yourself, then masturbate. If you feel uncertain as to whether you are sexually attracted to men or to women or to both, try to work it out before plunging into a confused sexual relationship. There are all sorts of groups that discuss sexuality and can be helpful to women with questions about their sexual orientation. There are also counselors and therapists who are skilled at helping women resolve sexual problems, and many women find it helpful to talk one-on-one. Sex should enhance a relationship and make the partners feel good about themselves; it should make them feel closer to each other.

ORGASM

Orgasm is the pinnacle of sexual release. Orgasmic response changes as you get older, and self-stimulation differs physiologically from sex with a partner. This is not to say that orgasm is better with or without a partner, or better at one age or another. But it *is* different, and your expectations should allow for these differences. During masturbation, orgasm is more intense but of briefer duration.

There has even been some recent information that distinguishes between a vaginal and a clitoral orgasm. While there are indeed women who reach orgasm without direct clitoral stimulation, this does not mean that it is a vaginal orgasm. There are few nerve endings in the vagina, so no woman should feel inadequate because she can only have an orgasm with clitoral stimulation. Biologically, orgasm happens the same way every time. It is of no importance to a woman how that orgasm is reached, and it doesn't matter where the stimulation comes from. What matters is how it *feels*. Some women can reach orgasm when their neck or earlobes are kissed; that does not mean we distinguish what type of orgasm it is.

The frequency of orgasm is also something that has been overemphasized in the media. A loving sexual encounter that leads to sexual satisfaction without orgasm is fine. There is no law stating that a woman must have an orgasm every time she makes love. However, if you find that you are frustrated by sex without orgasm, then it is a problem that should be resolved. Communication is key in attaining a sexually satisfying relationship. If you have trouble reaching an orgasm with a partner, guide him or her to stimulate you in a way you find erotically satisfying. Masturbation is a very useful practice for women who have difficulty reaching orgasm. Spend time privately exploring your body and discovering what physically stimulates you. It may be awkward at first, especially if you have been taught as a child that sex is dirty, but you should try to slowly work up to full sexual self-stimulation.

Multiple orgasm (one that goes on and on) is another recent focus of books and TV programs. Still, not many people really know what it is or if they have ever experienced it. In any case, no one can say whether multiple orgasm is better than one explosive orgasm. The key here is sexual satisfaction. Multiple orgasm is great if you have it, but no one has to have one. Women who have one satisfying orgasm are just as sexually fulfilled. Besides, many women don't reach orgasm during intercourse. This does not mean there is anything wrong with them; they just find sexual satisfaction in different ways. The hype about multiple orgasm is ridiculous; there is no need to label or quantify sexual release.

ORAL SEX

Oral sex is the stimulation of the genitals by a partner's mouth. When this is done to a woman, it is called cunnilingus. When it is performed on a man, it is called fellatio. Oral sex is a very common practice, and there are no reasons why it should be avoided. There is nothing dangerous or abnormal about it, and many people find it extremely satisfying. Oral sex is a choice, however, and a woman should not feel abnormal if she chooses not to participate in it. Remember that if you have more than one sexual partner, whether male or female, a dental dam (a protective sheet of latex or polyurethane) can help prevent the spread of STDs.

ANAL SEX

Anal sex, in which the anus rather than the vagina is penetrated, can be sexually pleasurable for some women. In many parts of the world, it is practiced as a means of birth control. However, many women find anal intercourse painful and not at all pleasurable. If you are one of those who finds anal sex unpleasant, you need not engage in it. There is a danger of tearing the rectal lining cells (mucosa) during anal penetration, because the tissue is very thin compared with that of the vagina. (Lubricating jellies can diminish the pain of anal intercourse.) Tearing of the mucosa can lead to an increase in the transmission of sexually transmitted diseases. The rectum does not have the natural protective barriers to disease that are present in the vaginal mucosa and its secretions. Also, vaginal or oral sex should never follow anal sex without first washing the penetrating object. Bacteria from the rectum can cause infection when introduced into the mouth or vagina.

With anal intercourse, infective organisms (bacteria and viruses) can be more easily transmitted into the bloodstream and are therefore more pathogenic (i.e., more capable of causing disease). Condoms offer some protection.

SEXUAL PROBLEMS

If you cannot enjoy sex, if you are fearful during sex, or if you are unable to comfortably stimulate yourself, there may be some psychological issues you need to address. These issues may range from fatigue or depression to a deeper psychological cause. A traumatic past sexual experience such as rape or incest can certainly be the cause of fear or anxiety during sex. Many times women have repressed the memory of such experiences as a defense mechanism, and they can't identify or resolve them without professional help. Often, fear or anxiety during sex is the only sign that a traumatic sexual experience occurred, and such a traumatic event should be investigated as a possible cause of sexual problems. You should see your health-care provider for a discussion about these possibilities, but note that not all medical providers are comfortable identifying or dealing with deep psychological problems. Nevertheless, the lack of enjoyment with sex is a problem, and if your health-care provider cannot help, you should ask for a reference for a qualified counselor or therapist.

Lack of sexual satisfaction may also reflect a problem with the relationship between two partners. It is difficult to enjoy sex with a partner who does not treat you well or with whom you have a poor emotional relationship. These issues are not to be taken lightly when trying to resolve sexual problems. Emotional and psychological issues are discussed in chapter 6.

Painful Sex

If you have had an episode of painful sex (dyspareunia), your next sexual encounter can be overlaid with anxiety ("Will it be painful again this time?"). Sexual response will be reduced and vaginal lubrication will be inadequate, thereby increasing the chances for another less-than-satisfying and even painful sexual encounter. It is important to interrupt this potentially disastrous cycle before it spirals out of control. For example, if the original pain was the result of a vaginal infection, get the infection treated. If the pain was a complication of a surgical procedure (episiotomy, hysterectomy, or labial biopsy, for example), give yourself more time to heal before engaging in the kind of sexual activity that will put stress on the surgical site. If the painful sexual experience involved rape, incest, or any nonconsensual act, intensive counseling may be necessary before sexual activity is resumed.

Once sex is finally resumed, an understanding sexual partner is an absolute requirement. All kinds of sexually stimulating activity may be attempted so long as it does not elicit pain. Go slowly; talk about what feels good and what may cause apprehension or pain. Don't even attempt vaginal penetration if you are afraid it may be painful. If and when you *are* ready, don't start with an erect penis or something of equivalent size. You might find vaginal dilators (graduated rubber dildos) useful, but you can also use your fingers.

Satisfying your personal sexual needs may require readjustments at different times in your life. Creativity and, if you have a partner, communication are the keys to attaining sexual satisfaction. Temporary states such as pregnancy will require adjustments in order to achieve sexual satisfaction. People with physical and mental disabilities have sexual needs and desires whose fulfillment may require mechanical aids or special therapy. As people get older, they may develop medical problems or may take medication that interferes with sexual response. This does not mean that sexual activity must end. In fact, this is a time when a communicative and creative sexual relationship becomes paramount. Find out what still feels good and what activities can enhance those feelings. If you are having trouble working out new elements in your sexual relationship, you may find help with an individual counselor, a couple's counselor, or a support group.

SEX IN THE TEENAGE YEARS

Sex among teenagers is becoming more and more commonplace. The incidence of teenage pregnancy in this country is staggering. According to estimates by the World Health Organization, the United States has the highest teenage pregnancy rate of any industrialized nation. Teenage women need to understand that sex is not something that happens *to* them; rather, it is an act that *they* decide to participate in. Women need to believe that they hold the power to determine what happens to their bodies. Teens should make a conscious decision to protect themselves from an unwanted pregnancy and from sexually transmitted diseases.

Unfortunately, educational programs promoting safer sex for teens have been shown to have little effect on their behavior. Even with the present threat of AIDS, many teenagers are not using condoms, even when they are readily available. Although a slight increase in regular condom usage was noted between 1990–1994, only 15 percent of heterosexually active teens use condoms regularly. (Regrettably, this percentage does not appreciably increase for older couples.) Although lesbians are at less risk of contracting STDs, during oral sex all women can use dental dams to reduce viral and bacterial transfer. Women need to take as much responsibility for their sexual activity as for any other area of their physical health.

SEX DURING THE TWENTIES AND THIRTIES

Generally, women in their twenties and thirties have a greater sense of control over their lives and bodies than teenagers do. Women of this age are responsible for their own health care and can readily obtain birth control. Sex is usually (but not always) a more conscious decision. However, women who decide not to engage in sexual activity at this age may be made to feel like social outcasts. Some choose to masturbate as a way to address their physical needs without risking pregnancy, STDs, or a psychological commitment to a partner.

Choosing celibacy at this age is perfectly acceptable, but being in a celibate relationship is a mutual decision on the part of two partners who communicate effectively. Sexual frustration in a relationship can be a very destructive force if both partners don't agree. A decision to remain celibate should not deny that there are strong sexual needs and desires that are very healthy and necessary. Masturbation, either solitary or mutual, can be a satisfying alternative to intercourse. Other activities such as physical exercise may cool the heat of the moment, but they are not ways to effectively deal with the emotions that result from denying normal sexual urges.

In a sexual relationship, there are often questions about what is the "normal" frequency for sex. Couples who live apart may engage in sex every time they are together. Then, as they live together (whether they are married or not), the frequency tapers off. Sex is different for each couple, and it must be emphasized that there is no "normal" frequency for sex. Frequency depends on mutual desire. If each partner is happy with sex once a week or once a month, that is perfectly normal. If couples want and enjoy sex every night, that is normal, too. Frequency becomes a problem only when it is not agreed upon; for example, when one partner wants sex more often than the other does. When this is the case, it takes respectful communication and commitment to work out an agreeable solution.

During the childbearing years, a woman's desire for sex may diminish. When caring for young children, both partners may be too tired for frequent sex. Accept this as normal, and know that frequency may increase as you move on to the next stage of life.

SEX IN THE FORTIES AND FIFTIES

If you are involved in a monogamous relationship, sex after age 40 can be better than it ever was before. You've learned what is pleasing for you and your partner, and you are comfortable with each other. Children are less physically demanding; they may even be grown and gone, and you have the time and the privacy to rekindle sexual excitement. That is the ideal scenario.

However, lots of women in this age group are starting new relationships following a divorce, separation, or widowhood and are facing sex with a new partner. Although starting over may make you feel young again, it can also be unsettling. It may bring a flood of feelings of insecurity resembling those of the teenage years.

As you approach menopause, your body naturally changes contour. Traditionally, women in this age group are insecure about their bodies, having gained some weight since childbearing years, and they may not feel they live up to a certain ideal of sexual attractiveness. The solution to the problem of feeling eternally "sexy" lies not in trying to regain that 18-year-old body but rather in learning to accept a normal body of a 40- or 50-year-old. Positive body image and self-esteem are sexy.

SEX AFTER MENOPAUSE

Sex in the postmenopausal years is a very healthful activity. Sex is good for you, as it keeps the vaginal tissue healthy and moist and delays the genitals' aging process. Sexual response is different after menopause, but still enjoyable. If you have a sexual partner, it is critical to discuss how your sexual needs and responses have changed so that those needs can be met. If you or your partner has recently had a heart attack or any other medical problem, discuss with your health-care provider and your partner any limitations the two of you may have in your physical activity, including sex. It's common for a sexually active heart attack survivor to worry about dying during orgasm. You may also feel a decrease in sexual desire after menopause. Discuss this issue with your partner, and see how you can resolve it to mutual satisfaction. You should also talk to your health-care provider, since hormone replacement therapy may help restore some of the loss in libido.

The entire decision-making process about sex will change after menopause. There is no longer the risk of an unwanted pregnancy, but the risk of sexually transmitted diseases still exists. If you are embarking on a new sexual relationship, the use of condoms to protect against disease is still crucial.

3

THE GYNECOLOGICAL (GYN) EXAM

There are many reasons why a woman should go to a gynecological health-care provider. The most common reasons women seek the advice of their gynecologist, gyn nurse-practitioner, or midwife are to address a specific problem, to get routine preventive care, or to obtain contraceptives. Don't let the word "routine" be misleading. Each visit for preventive care should be personalized and meet the special needs of each woman. Every woman should be comfortable with her own body, but each woman has different needs and comfort levels. An important part of the gynecological health-care professional's role is to promote that comfort, answer questions, and provide information.

A woman who seeks gynecological care is not merely a collection of reproductive and sexual organs. When you go for a gynecological (gyn) exam, you should expect to detail your entire medical, family, and social history so that your caregiver can understand your individual needs. Many issues, such as a history of incest, past or ongoing domestic violence, loss of libido, inability to attain an orgasm, urinary incontinence, fear of cancer, or uncertainty about body parts and functions, can be difficult to bring up to your health-care provider. Difficult as these topics may be to discuss, your provider is someone who is trained to help you deal with them and make you feel comfortable with your own body. A thorough gynecological history should include questions on these topics, but if your provider doesn't ask specifically, be clear that you need to discuss them. It is the caregiver's role to open as many doors as possible so that you can feel comfortable talking about all areas of your health.

Women often use their gynecological health-care practitioners as their primary health-care providers. This is fine as long as these women don't have any underlying medical problems and as long as the gynecologist is aware of and has training in medical areas other than the reproductive system. Young women often switch from a pediatrician to a gynecologist when they are considering becoming sexually active. They often have no other medical problems for many years, so their gynecologist, nurse-practitioner, or nurse-midwife takes care of most, if not all, of their medical needs.

Good gynecological health depends on good medical and mental health. Proper nutrition, exercise, avoidance of tobacco and other addictive substances, safer sex, and sexual responsibility are all part of optimal health. If you have any questions or problems in these areas, feel free to discuss them during your first gyn exam and at every visit thereafter. The gyn exam should be a learning experience for a woman, not a traumatic event. It can be an opportunity to learn how to do a breast self-exam and to understand the importance of it. The pelvic exam is a great opportunity to learn more about how your body works.

WHY GO

What makes a woman seek gynecological care? What issues should a woman consider appropriate for her gynecological health-care provider? First and foremost, women need not have a physical or psychological problem to seek gynecological care. Many women unconsciously feel they don't deserve the luxury of having a preventive exam. But the more they get routine preventive care, the fewer problems will result. Think of it like getting your teeth examined and cleaned. The more regularly you do it, generally the fewer the dental problems.

If you do have a gynecological problem, it can center on several different issues: menstrual problems (delayed onset of menstruation, loss of periods, or irregular, painful, heavy, or unusually light periods); sexuality (heterosexuality, lesbianism, bisexuality, and celibacy; libido and sexual response; fear of sex and the concomitant issues of incest, sexual abuse, and rape); sexual satisfaction (orgasm, masturbation, pain during or after sex); safer sex and sexual responsibility; or reproductive issues (contraception, conception, fertility and infertility, family planning, pregnancy, abortion, miscarriage, ectopic pregnancy, and the biological time clock).

Changes in physical or mental outlook associated with menopause and aging should also be a topic of discussion with your gyn provider. The detection and prevention of cancer, and the fear of cancer, are relevant health-care issues. Infections of the breast, vagina, and pelvic organs should be examined promptly. Breast lumps, sudden or severe pain, or bleeding should also be investigated without delay.

You should be able to bring a wide range of problems to the attention of your gynecological health-care provider. You may want to bring up a problem at your routine exam or make a special appointment to discuss a specific problem. For instance, decreased interest in sex may be ongoing and something to discuss at your annual exam. But if your relationship is seriously threatened because of it, you will want to see your practitioner right away. You needn't be made to feel that any issue is irrelevant or inconsequential, and you should expect a thorough, careful, and caring response along with appropriate treatment or proper referral for care.

WHOM TO GO TO

Who provides proper gynecological care? Nurses with specific training and expertise in gynecology include gyn nurse-practitioners and certified nurse-midwives. Nurse-midwives also provide full obstetrical care. These advanced-practice nurses are skilled at screening for problems and providing preventive care. They also tend to spend more time instructing their patients. If these nurses detect problems that require medical training or surgical skills, they immediately confer with their consulting physicians.

All physicians get some training in gynecology, and some family physicians and internists expand and hone their training so that they remain skilled in providing women's health care. Obstetrician/gynecologists are specially trained in women's health care and in the management of pregnancy, labor, and delivery. Some obstetricians specialize in maternal-fetal medicine (also called high-risk obstetrics) and limit their care to women with complicated pregnancies. Some gynecologists give up obstetrical practice and provide women's health care only to nonpregnant women. Some gynecologists subspecialize: gynecological oncologists care only for women with gynecological cancers; gynecological endocrinologists care only for women with fertility or hormonal problems. Your health-care provider should know his or her own capabilities and limitations and should refer you to a more specialized practitioner when necessary.

THE OVERALL EXAM

What's involved in the gyn exam? Your gynecological exam should be informative and straightforward. Your practitioner should make you comfortable; if he or she does not, choose another practitioner who can meet your emotional and medical needs. If it's your first exam, try not to focus on the horror stories that your friend, sister, mother, or grandmother might have told you. If you've had a previous bad experience, tell your new practitioner so that he or she can be even more sensitive to your needs. If he or she lacks sensitivity, choose a different practitioner.

A visit to the gynecological health-care provider should never, under any circumstances, be imbued with sexual innuendo, sexual overtones, or sexual advances. This is a medical setting, and any sexual inferences by the caregiver are totally inappropriate. If you feel that your provider has crossed his or her professional boundaries, point it out to him or her. If the provider doesn't cease the behavior at once, get up and leave. Do not hesitate to spread the word about this type of practitioner or to press charges if he or she crosses the boundary of legal behavior. You should feel absolutely safe in the care of your gyn health-care provider. If you are uncomfortable in the exam room alone with your practitioner, request that a third party be present for the exam. Some states require that a female nurse or physician's assistant (PA) be present during a pelvic exam. You should also feel that everything you say is confidential, unless you authorize your caregiver to discuss it with others. This includes parents, spouses, and partners.

When you go to any health-care provider for the first time, make certain ground rules clear. If you wish to be addressed by your first name, by a nickname, or by your last name and a particular title, inform your health-care provider and his or her staff. Ask your provider how he or she wishes to be addressed. Introductions such as "Hello, Nancy, I'm Dr. Smith" are demeaning and are not acceptable, even though you may later establish that you wish to be addressed by your first name and you wish to address your health-care provider by a last name and title. Your first encounter with your health-care provider should take place in an office while you are fully clothed. Don't allow yourself to be herded into an examination room to get undressed before you've gotten a chance to meet your health-care provider and fully discussed all the issues you've set out to cover. (Unless, of course, your health-care provider wishes to take your history while you are *both* wearing only skimpy examination gowns, thereby equalizing your positions.) After you are shown into the examination room, you should be given an adequate amount of time to undress in privacy. If on subsequent visits you wish to discuss a particular matter with your practitioner, make sure that his or her staff understands you would like some consultation time (while you are fully clothed). If you prefer to get your exam completed quickly, you may choose to have your visit take place entirely in the exam room. Remember, the choice should be yours.

Although most women don't look forward to a gynecological examination, the gyn exam should never be traumatic or painful. If any part of the exam becomes unbearable, have your caregiver stop at once. You may need some time to regroup emotionally, or you may find that part of the exam will have to be deferred to another visit. If this is the case, some investigation should be done to identify why the exam was so uncomfortable. Whether it is a physical problem that is causing pain or the memories of abusive behavior, your caregiver should respect your needs and help you deal with the situation. Most caregivers can suggest ways (such as breathing techniques) to help you get through the emotional and physical difficulties of the exam. You should feel comfortable working through these issues with your caregiver; if you find yourself in an adversarial position with your healthcare provider, change providers.

The exam itself should be thorough, educational, and not unpleasant. The exam table's head should be slightly elevated so you can have eye contact with the practitioner throughout the exam. The exam should include such basics as a blood pressure check, a general inspection of the skin (with reminders to reduce sun exposure), and, when appropriate, a temperature check. You should expect your thyroid gland to be felt, because thyroid abnormalities are common in women. (The thyroid is located in the middle of the neck just below the Adam's apple.) If you do not have an internist, your practitioner may also check your eyes, throat, and teeth. You should expect your lungs and heart to be listened to with a stethoscope.

The Breast Exam

The next part of the exam should include a thorough breast exam. This is the time to learn the technique and importance of breast self-examination and to ask about breast self-exam pamphlets and other teaching aids. Some of these brochures are designed as patient reminders to be placed at home in the medicine chest or dressing area. Plastic-coated brochures can be hung right in the shower, and your care provider should have some to give you. Once you feel confident doing a breast self-exam, expect your examiner to proceed to the abdominal exam. But don't allow the examiner to go on if you still have questions about the breast exam: You have the right to ask questions until you clearly understand.

The Abdominal Exam

The entire belly should be inspected for any skin problems and for hair distribution patterns. Your examiner will then apply gentle pressure to feel your abdominal organs (e.g., liver and spleen) for any enlargements or abnormalities. This may bother you if you are very ticklish, but it should not be painful.

The Pelvic Exam

The examination of the pelvic organs then follows. A sheet should be provided for the gyn exam. If one is not offered, ask for it. The sheet should cover your genitals until you are in the most comfortable position possible, with your feet in the stirrups of the exam table. You should be encouraged to relax your inner thigh muscles, thus allowing your legs to drop apart as if your knees were trying to touch opposite walls. Or the inner thigh muscles can be gently touched to show which muscles need to relax in order to make the exam more comfortable. Both of these maneuvers should be done while your genitals are still covered. A caregiver should never abruptly expose your genitals, nor should he or she push your legs apart. Both actions are violations.

Once you are relatively comfortable, the caregiver should announce that he or she is going to push back the sheet so that the external genitals can be carefully inspected. The examiner should warn you before he or she touches you. The first touch should be on a relatively exposed place, such as the upper leg, then the external genital area, and then the area just inside the vagina. Next the inside of the vagina and the cervix are to be examined with a warmed speculum. Your practitioner should explain all of these steps beforehand.

The Pap Smear

The Pap smear (a slide test that can differentiate normal from abnormal cells) should then be performed. The Pap smear detects abnormalities of the cervix. It is a safe, noninvasive test for cervical cancer, an easily treatable form of cancer when detected early. Cervical cancer occurs in older and younger women alike but is uncommon in those who have never been heterosexually active. Since this screening test is so simple and relatively inexpensive, there is no good reason not to have it done on an annual basis.

Your caregiver should tell you that he or she will be using one or two swablike instruments before scraping your cervix with them. (Some women find that their cervices are very sensitive to touch, and all women should be forewarned before cervical manipulation.) The Pap smear is obtained by gathering cells from inside the cervical canal and from the outside rim of the cervix. The instruments used to obtain a Pap smear are a tiny soft brush resembling a miniature bottle brush and a small spatula resembling a popsicle stick. Some practitioners use an instrument that combines these two instruments. Sometimes the Pap smear can cause light spotting (bleeding), especially in pregnant women, and your examiner should warn you of this possibility. Spotting is not abnormal, though, and in cases of infection or severe inflammation, the amount of bleeding may be greater. If you have come in complaining of symptoms of a vaginal infection or if you want to be tested for gonorrhea or chlamydia, a sample of cells can be obtained for testing at the time the Pap smear is obtained. If you want to see your cervix, this is also the time to ask for a mirror and have your provider point out your anatomy. The speculum should then be gently removed.

The examiner must then thoroughly feel the outline of the uterus, fallopian tubes, and ovaries. This is done by carefully inserting one or two fingers of a gloved hand into the vagina and pushing firmly yet gently up on the cervix while the other hand is pushing firmly yet gently downward on the lower abdomen. This may sound uncomfortable, but the exam should not be painful if it is done properly. If you tighten your abdominal wall muscles, your examiner will have to push down with greater force and might not get as much information as necessary. Therefore, you should be as relaxed as possible so that you don't involuntarily tighten your abdominal muscles.

The Rectal Exam

The rectal exam is the final part of the gynecologic exam. Using one well-lubricated finger in the vagina and a second well-lubricated finger in the rectum, your examiner can best feel any uterine or ovarian abnormalities. In addition, the lowest third of the rectum can be checked for abnormal masses, and the stool can be checked for blood. Both of these tests are extremely important in all women over 40 years of age. Nobody enjoys the rectal exam, but if you breathe slowly and keep your abdominal muscles relaxed, the exam can be quick and bearable.

Summing Up

Your caregiver should help you sit up, give you a little time to collect yourself, and then allow time for you to ask any questions about the exam or visit. Be aware that most physicians schedule a gyn exam into a 15-minute time slot. This does not leave much time for discussion of complicated issues. Nurse-midwives who are taught to focus on patient instruction often schedule 30 to 45 minutes for a gyn exam, and sometimes even longer. It is helpful for patients to realize this ahead of time when booking the appointment. The complaint that patients most often have about their gyn visits is that they feel rushed. If you know you'll need more time to address your issues, ask to be scheduled for the amount of time necessary or make a follow-up appointment. Neither you nor your caregiver should feel rushed. The gyn exam should not be intimidating; it should be informative and empowering.

It should demystify a woman's sexual organs and functions. It should allow women to feel comfortable with themselves. In a society where many television and advertising images are suffused with sexual innuendo but where sexual education and explicit sexual discussion are not universally acceptable, the visit to the gynecological health-care provider can and should be a liberating and enlightening experience.

4

$\mathcal{C}$ONTRACEPTION

*W*hen a woman makes the choice to become sexually active with a man, there are products available that can allow them the freedom of choosing whether and when they would like to have children. Responsible people who engage in sex must consider the long-term health consequences of the act. These include each partner's emotional commitment to the other, a concerted effort to reduce the chances of spreading sexually transmitted diseases, and a mutual decision to avoid an unplanned pregnancy. Heretofore, the responsibility for contraception has been handed almost exclusively to women.

The issue of contraception in the United States is a complicated one. Because this very important health issue has been turned into a political hot potato, contraceptive choices have been limited and the encouragement of contraceptive research has been severely diminished. Women and children are bearing the brunt of the medicolegal and political infighting that pervade our country's approach to health issues. There are more than 3 million unplanned pregnancies in the United States every year and more than 1 million of these occur among teenagers. In the next decade, the earth's population will increase by a number equal to the entire population living on the planet in 1800. These stunning facts should be the very impetus that propels the political and scientific communities to join together to restore this country to the forefront of contraceptive research.

In addition, the public must make clear to scientists as well as government officials that it wants a wider range of safe contraceptive choices. In so doing, people must be willing to frankly discuss sex, family planning, sexual practices, and the birth control options that best address their needs. The scientific community and pharmaceutical industry must realize that there is public support for improving the range of contraceptive choices. Although there will never be a "perfect" contraceptive that will suit every couple's needs, the goal should be a wider array of choices that offer the greatest contraceptive benefits with the least possible health risks. Pregnancy poses certain risks to a woman's health, and any birth control method should pose a lesser health risk than pregnancy. Sex, like pregnancy, is not risk-free. If we expect intensive contraceptive research from the scientific community, then we cannot thwart that effort by expecting contraceptive products to be risk-free. Safe, yes; but risk-free is simply not possible.

Besides safety, the other major contraceptive issue is effectiveness. It is extremely important to understand how a birth control method's effectiveness in preventing pregnancy is determined. Some statistical references are based on theoretical rates of contraceptive potential—i.e., the ideal rate of contraception if the method is used properly 100 percent of the time. Other effectiveness rates are based on user rates—i.e., the actual rate of contraception as determined by the actual use of a particular method. User rates sound more realistic, but one must be careful to include in those user rates only those people who attempt to use a particular method faithfully. One should not include individuals for whom contraceptives were prescribed but who have failed to use them actively, such as a woman who is fitted for a diaphragm but who either never buys it or never uses it. If you want to compare how effective one birth control method is to another, you must use the same statistical evaluation. The particular statistical method used to calculate the effectiveness rate is of less importance than the use of a consistent method.

CURRENT CONTRACEPTIVE CHOICES

Barrier Contraception

Barrier methods are those that mechanically and/or chemically block the progression of sperm as they pass through a woman's cervix on their way to fertilize an ovum. Barrier contraceptives include spermicides, condoms, diaphragms, cervical caps, the contraceptive sponge, and the recently approved female condom.

Spermicides. Spermicides are chemical agents that immobilize and destroy sperm. Currently, there are only two FDA-approved spermicides available: nonoxynol-9 and octocynol-9. Nonoxynol-9 is the spermicidal agent most commonly found in the majority of American spermicides. Their modes of action are similar, and they are contained in various preparations—creams, foams, gels, suppositories, soluble film, dissolvable tablets, etc. The only difference among these products is the amount of time it takes them to become active and to remain active. Their effectiveness ranges from 80 to 85 percent when used consistently. That efficacy increases when the spermicide is held against the cervix with a cervical cap or diaphragm, or when the spermicide is used in conjunction with a male condom or a female condom.

Spermicides are relatively easy to obtain, since they can be purchased at local pharmacies and some convenience stores without a prescription. The cost will vary slightly from store to store, but each package ranges from about $6.50 for suppositories to $10.50 for foam, which makes the cost per use about $.75 to $1. Spermicides have relatively few risks, the main one being a sensitivity or allergy to the product that can cause vaginal or vulval irritation and/or burning.

Spermicides also tend to be a bit messy, which is a problem for some couples.

Condoms. Condoms are one of the oldest forms of birth control. They are a thin covering that sheathes the penis and collects the ejaculated sperm. The condom is unrolled and stretched over the erect penis prior to any penile ejaculation. Originally, condoms were made from animal bladders or sheep intestines. Animal, or "natural," condoms are still available. They tend to be thinner than latex condoms, and therefore interfere less with penile sensitivity, but they are more expensive. Latex condoms are more widely available and more widely used. They are inexpensive and come in different sizes and styles (smooth or ribbed, with or without a reservoir tip, lubricated or nonlubricated, for example). More important, they offer protection from the passage of sperm, bacteria, and viruses. Latex condoms play an important role in the attempt to reduce the spread of sexually transmitted diseases, including gonorrhea, herpes, hepatitis, and AIDS. Natural-skin condoms are more porous and may allow the passage of bacteria and viruses, though they prevent the passage of sperm.

By using condoms that contain a spermicide, or by including spermicide or vaginal contraceptive sponges in regular condom use, you can increase the condom's effectiveness rate in pregnancy prevention and possibly in STD control (although the effectiveness of spermicide in preventing disease is now being debated). When consistently used with spermicide, condoms offer greater than 90 percent efficacy in preventing unplanned pregnancy. However, by adding oil-based lubricants such as baby oil or petroleum jelly, the latex will begin to deteriorate within minutes, thus destroying its ability to prevent pregnancy or STDs. If a condom breaks or slips off during intercourse, call your practitioner within twenty-four hours for the "Morning after" pill. (See page 52.)

The cost of condoms now ranges between $.50 to $1.00 each for latex condoms and $3.50 to $4.50 each for natural-skin condoms. Condoms, especially the latex variety, are widely available and can now be purchased almost anywhere, including pharmacies, grocery stores, gas stations, and even some restaurant rest rooms. They are sometimes distributed free of charge at many family planning clinics.

Diaphragms.   Diaphragms have been available in the United States for almost a century, thanks to the pioneering efforts of women's contraceptive rights advocates led by Margaret Sanger. A diaphragm is a shallow latex disk that serves as a receptacle for spermicide and as a barrier against sperm, and *it should always be used with a spermicide.* The diaphragm has a flexible rim. Prior to insertion, the diaphragm is folded in half, then slipped into the vagina behind the pubic bone to cover the cervix. When properly inserted into the vagina, the diaphragm holds the spermicide against the cervix, thereby preventing the passage of sperm on its path toward the ovum. Before using your diaphragm, always check for holes or cracks in the latex. If you find that the diaphragm is damaged, you must use alternative birth control measures until you replace it.

The diaphragm comes in varying sizes, from 50 to 105 millimeters in diameter, and with varying spring construction of its rim so that most women can be easily fitted. Proper fit by a health-care professional is essential. A diaphragm that is too small can slip from its position covering the cervix as the upper vagina expands during orgasm, and it may also be painful as it moves around. A diaphragm that is too large can bend or slip during intercourse, leaving the cervix uncovered. A large diaphragm can be uncomfortable for the user and often for her partner as well. In addition, a diaphragm that is too large puts greater pressure on the urethra and consequently can further increase the risk of urinary tract infection. A properly fitted diaphragm rests behind the pubic bone and puts some pressure on the urethra, and this may be one of the factors associated with a small increased risk of urinary tract infection in diaphragm users.

Like all barrier methods of birth control, the diaphragm must be put into place with spermicide before intercourse takes place. It may be inserted up to eight hours prior to coitus, and it must be left in place at least six hours after coitus. It is thought that additional spermicide should be inserted into the vagina (without removing the diaphragm) with each act of coitus; however, this is controversial as well as messy. There is some evidence, albeit poor, to show that two successive acts of intercourse less than six hours apart must be preceded by additional jelly. This advice originated with the distributors of spermicidal jelly, who, of course, want you to use more of their product.

You should never remove a diaphragm until you are sure that six hours have elapsed since the last act of intercourse. Putting an extra applicator full of jelly in before the six-hour limit is optional, but after six hours it is absolutely necessary. It must be remembered that the diaphragm itself is *not* a contraceptive; it is a receptacle for contraceptive cream or jelly. Like an umbrella frame without any cloth, a diaphragm by itself offers minimal protection. When used properly, the diaphragm provides more than a 90 percent efficacy rate.

The most common reason for the failure of the diaphragm is failure to insert it. The diaphragm does not work in the bureau drawer. In the heat of passion it's easy to rationalize that it is not worth inserting. This happens more frequently with women who feel the need for privacy in completing the insertion. Compliance rates increase dramatically when diaphragm insertion becomes part of sexual foreplay. There is nothing wrong with teaching your partner to insert the diaphragm. That way it can be done just before intercourse and not interfere with oral sex.

A major advantage of the diaphragm is its ability to hold menstrual blood during menses. This can make sex during your period substantially less messy.

The diaphragm has relatively few health risks. You may have a slightly increased risk of urinary tract infection, especially if the diaphragm is ill-fitting. There is the remote risk of toxic shock syndrome (TSS) associated with any device inserted and left in the vagina, but the incidence of TSS involving diaphragm use is very low. Otherwise, the diaphragm poses the same risks that spermicides do: allergy or sensitivity.

The cost of a diaphragm is about $20, and the device should be replaced every year or two, depending on how often it is used. You will also have to pay for an office visit to your practitioner for a fitting. Your practitioner will give you a prescription for an appropriately

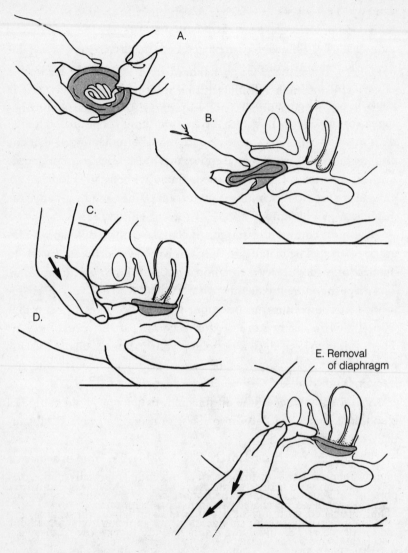

Figure 4.1. Inserting the Diaphragm

sized diaphragm, and the actual purchase is made at a pharmacy. The spermicidal cream or jelly is an extra cost.

Contraceptive sponge. The contraceptive sponge was widely available until 1994. It was temporarily removed from the market because of problems maintaining a manufacturing milieu low in bacteria. As of this printing, manufacture has not yet resumed, and the current manufacturer has no plans to do so.

The sponge is a spermicide-impregnated piece of polyurethane. It is 2¼ inches in diameter and ¾ inch thick. It can be used by any woman and need not be fitted for size. The sponge is simple to use: Just moisten it and place it in the upper vagina. It can be left safely in place for up to 24 hours. Like a diaphragm, it may be inserted several hours before intercourse, and it has a string attached to its underside so that it can easily be removed. Although the contraceptive sponge works like a diaphragm—by placing a high concentration of spermicide against the cervix—it is not individually fitted and therefore has a greater chance of slipping from its cervical position, particularly in women who have had at least one child. The vagina does not have as much tone once a woman has given birth, so there is more room and the sponge can slip. Consequently, the sponge's efficacy is less than the diaphragm's: about 85 percent for women who have never had a baby and about 71 percent for women who have delivered a baby. The sponge's effectiveness can be increased to 90 percent if the male partner uses a condom.

In the past, contraceptive sponges could be obtained at a pharmacy and cost about $9 for a package of six. You did not need to have a physical exam for a fitting, so the cost of an office visit was eliminated. Sponges could be purchased without a prescription.

The pregnancy risk for sponge users was approximately 20 percent, with a higher rate for women who had already had a vaginal delivery. In some women, there was also the risk of allergy or sensitivity to the spermicide. As with other vaginal barrier methods, a slightly elevated risk of toxic shock syndrome with sponge use had been reported.

Cervical caps. The cervical cap was approved for usage by the U.S. Food and Drug Administration (FDA) in 1988. This is a small

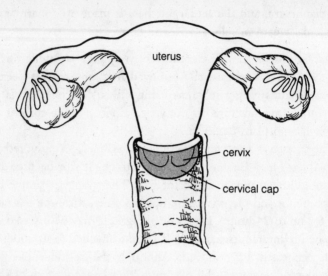

Figure 4.2. Proper Fit of a Cervical Cap

latex cup that fits snugly over the cervix and works much the same way as the diaphragm in blocking sperm from the cervical opening. The cap may be left in place for 48 hours, making it more acceptable for some barrier contraceptive users. As with a diaphragm, it is recommended that you insert extra spermicide into the vagina for added protection should you have intercourse several times within those 48 hours. Because the cervical cap does not place any pressure against the urethra, there is not an associated increase in the risk of urinary tract infections. Unfortunately, the cervical cap is available only in four different sizes, and some women are unable to be fitted. The cap itself, which resembles a thimble with a wide rim, should be used with a spermicide. The spermicide is placed into the cap, and the rim fits over the cervix. To insert the cap, use your fingers to place it over the cervix. Because the cap must be placed snugly over the cervix, some women find it difficult or even impossible to insert one properly. Removing the cap involves using your finger to break the seal between the cap and the cervix and then pulling the cap out of the vagina. Unlike the contraceptive sponge, the cervical cap does not have a string attached for easy re-

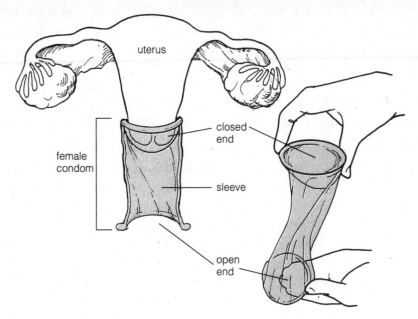

Figure 4.3. Female Condom

moval. To avoid damage to the cervix, it is important that first the suction be broken and then the cap be gently removed.

Cervical caps must be fitted by a qualified health-care provider. Many health-care providers have never been taught how to fit cervical caps; consequently, they do not offer caps to their patients. Caps are best fitted when a woman is at midcycle in her menstrual period. Any cap should be rechecked for proper fit after any occurrence that affects the cervix, including labor, abortion, miscarriage, dilation and curettage (D&C), or cervical treatment with freezing, burning, or laser.

Although initial evaluations reported a higher incidence of abnormal Pap smears in cervical cap users, more recent and extensive studies in the late 1980s have not corroborated this finding. Cervical caps are not recommended for use during menses because of the remotely increased risk of toxic shock syndrome. Moreover, they should not be used by women with abnormal Pap smears or by women with cervical, vaginal, or pelvic infections.

The cervical cap costs more than a diaphragm, and you may have a difficult time finding a provider who offers them in certain localities. The cost of the cap is about $40, and the additional fee for a fitting by your health-care provider is approximately $65 to $80. If the cap is a contraceptive device that appeals to you, before making an appointment call and ask your health-care provider if he or she offers it. If not, he or she might be able to refer you to someone who does.

Female condoms.   The so-called female condom was developed to reduce the spread of sexually transmitted diseases that can occur when the outside of the vagina comes into contact with the scrotum and base of the penis. The female condom is a malleable, tube-shaped pouch of polyurethane or latex with a flexible polyurethane ring at either end. Spermicide can be placed on the cervix side of the inner ring (as with the diaphragm) for extra protection, and this inner ring is inserted into the vagina. The outer ring (the larger side) is then placed over the labia. During intercourse the penis pushes the inner ring against the cervix, eliminating the need to have a precise cervical fit. The female condom can be obtained through family planning clinics and through pharmacies.

Studies in Western Europe, where it has been commercially released for some time, show efficacy comparable to the male condom in preventing pregnancy and STDs.

Oral Contraceptive Pills

The Pill became commercially available in the United States in 1960. Although it revolutionized the birth control options available, over the succeeding years its popularity has waxed and waned. These fluctuations in oral contraceptive use have reflected media focus on the most recent findings about the Pill's risks and effectiveness. During these years, the actual hormonal content of the Pill has been decreased, thereby reducing medical complications and unpleasant side effects associated with the original formulation. However, because of the public perception of the Pill as a high-risk birth control method, Pill use is actually less than it was two decades ago.

The Pill is made up of a combination of synthetic hormones that mimic the effects of natural estrogen and progesterone. Normally these hormones stimulate ovulation, but oral contraceptives are prepared in a formula that simulates pregnancy and blocks ovulation. In combination, they affect the areas of the brain that normally stimulate the ovary to produce ova ("eggs"). In addition, these hormones reduce the production of cervical mucus, which normally aids the course of sperm into the uterus, and they cause a thinning of the uterine lining. This thinning provides a poor environment for the implantation of an ovum and reduces monthly bleeding.

The Pill is taken every day for three weeks. During the fourth week no pills are taken, or they are replaced with inactive reminder ("dummy") pills. Bleeding will occur during the fourth week—two or three days after the last oral contraceptive has been taken. This bleeding is usually lighter than a normal period, and sometimes after long-term use of the Pill it may diminish to almost nothing. Decreased monthly bleeding reduces a woman's chances of becoming anemic and is one of the advantages of birth control pills. The disappearance of monthly bleeding, while not medically dangerous, may make some women worry that they could be pregnant. If monthly flow stops altogether, a different Pill formulation can be tried so that some flow occurs for those women who prefer monthly bleeding. It should be noted that this bleeding is not a menstrual period but a "withdrawal bleed"—a pharmacological outcome of the withdrawal of the Pill's hormones during the fourth week. If the Pill's hormonal effects on the uterine lining are extremely effective in preventing cellular buildup, there will be no bleeding when the hormones are withdrawn. Again, this is not a problem. If you take your pills daily, the chance that you will get pregnant is almost nil. But if a monthly bleed is a source of reassurance, or if it makes you feel more normal, a different type of Pill can be tried.

The oral contraceptives currently on the market have very low amounts of both estrogen and progesterone. When the Pill first became available three decades ago, it had about three times more estrogen in it than it generally does today. Also, those higher-dose pills caused more side effects, such as nausea and headache, and were associated with an increased risk of serious complications, such as blood clots and stroke. Undoubtedly, the risk of serious medical complications is enormously increased in Pill takers over age 35 who smoke. In fact, older studies suggesting that birth control pills can increase the risk of death from stroke, heart attack, or blood clots have been shown to be invalid for nonsmoking, low-dose Pill users who are pre-meno-pausal.

As far as side effects are concerned, low-dose pills can initially cause slight nausea and headache, which almost always spontaneously disappear within the first, second, or third cycle. Spotting or very irregular bleeding, also known as breakthrough bleeding, is a common complaint, but this too clears up by the third or fourth cycle. Bloating, acne, and minor weight gain (three to five pounds) are not unusual problems in women who use the Pill. These side effects may diminish over time as well. Every woman reacts differently to the hormonal combinations of various oral contraceptives. One particular brand may suit her best, but because most side effects resolve themselves by the end of the third cycle, it is not advisable to switch brands before giving the present one at least a three-month trial. Combination oral contraceptive pills should not be taken by women who have just begun to breast-feed, because the estrogen in the Pill can suppress lactation. But after about three months, when a stable lactation pattern has been established, low-dose combination oral contraceptive pills are safe and do not interfere with milk production.

The Pill must be taken once a day, preferably at about the same time each day. This is especially important now because of the reduced levels of hormones in today's low-dose pills. With this low level of hormones, if you are even a few hours late taking your pill, you may bleed a bit (breakthrough bleeding). If you forget to take one, you lose some of the Pill's ability to suppress ovulation, and your risk of pregnancy is increased. If you should ever forget to take your pill, take it as soon as you remember and be sure to follow it with the next one at your regular time. This may mean you are taking two pills at once; there is nothing wrong with doing that, but you may feel a bit nauseated afterward. To be on the safe side, you should use an additional method of birth control, like a condom, until the end of that particular cycle. If you take the Pill every single day without fail, it offers more than a 99.5 percent rate of contraception.

Over the years, the Pill, along with several environmental factors, has been linked by some to female cancers. To date, no large studies have shown the Pill to be a cancer-causing agent. Although the Pill has not been shown to be a causative factor in cervical cancer, there is an increased rate of cervical cancer and precancerous changes among Pill users. And cervical cancer is also more common in women with multiple sexual partners. Whether this indicates that Pill users tend to have multiple sexual partners is unclear.

Endometrial (uterine lining) cancer is actually shown to be almost 50 percent less common in women who have taken the Pill. This protective effect increases with the use and continues for an unknown length of time after oral contraceptives are discontinued. A similar protective effect is seen with ovarian cancer. In women who have taken the Pill, there seems to be about a 40-50 percent reduction in ovarian cancer, and protection increases with longer use. Again, the protection continues for an unknown length of time even after the Pill is discontinued. Although almost every environmental agent under the sun, including the Pill, has been linked at some time to the rising rate of breast cancer in the United States, no respected study has linked the Pill itself to an increased risk for developing breast cancer. In addition, Pill users have a much reduced rate of benign breast disease.

Currently, one of the Pill's major drawbacks is its cost. You must have a yearly office visit (at varying fees) in order to be examined and given the prescription. The pills are available only from a pharmacy and only by prescription. The price varies slightly according to brand and to your region of the United States, but the cost is generally between $16 and $26 per pack.

Progestin-only pills ("mini-pills"). Progestin-only birth control pills, also known as mini-pills, are available in the United States but are used much less frequently than combination pills. They are less popular because they offer less birth control protection (97 percent versus 99.5 percent in combination pills) and because they commonly cause very irregular bleeding. Because progestin-only pills have no estrogen to suppress lactation, they can be used by women who are breast-feeding. Estrogen is also associated with an increased risk of blood clots, so progestin-only pills can be a safer alternative for women who have had cardiovascular disease (i.e., heart attack and blood clots). They are taken every day of the year and include no week of placebo (inactive) pills. The "minipill" is more expensive than the combination pill, costing more than $35.

The morning-after pill.   Although there are currently no drugs specifically approved by the FDA to prevent pregnancy after unprotected intercourse, certain pill formulations can be used for this purpose. There is one widely available birth control pill that contains 50 micrograms of the estrogen ethinyl estradiol and 0.5 milligrams of the progestin norgestrel and is marketed under the trade name Ovral. Two pills should be taken as soon as possible after unprotected intercourse or contraceptive failure has occurred. The second dose of two pills must be taken 12 hours later. There is another birth control pill that may also be used. It contains 30 micrograms of ethinyl estradiol and 0.15 milligrams of levonorgestrel and is marketed under the trade names of Nordette or Levlen. Four of these pills must be taken as soon as possible and repeated twelve hours later. The pills must be started within 72 hours of intercourse, but preferably in the 12 to 24 hours following intercourse. After 72 hours, there is an increased chance of becoming pregnant. Studies have shown a pregnancy prevention rate from as low as 70 percent to as high as 98.2 percent with this regimen. The dosage of hormones in morning-after pills has been associated with breast tenderness, mild headache, nausea, and vomiting. If vomiting does occur within an hour, the dose should be repeated. If pregnancy occurs, there is a theoretical risk of fetal malformation, although none has been reported.

Levonorgestrel (*Norplant*)

The most recently developed hormonal contraceptive is levonorgestrel (commonly known by its brand name, *Norplant*). This device consists of six progestin-impregnated rods that are surgically inserted just below the skin of the upper arm. Each rod is less than an $^1/8$ inch in diameter and approximately $1^1/2$ inch long. The progestin in the rods is slowly released over the five-year life span of the device. The contraceptive action of synthetic progesterone is based on its ability to thin out and even atrophy the lining of the uterus, create thickened cervical mucus (which makes it difficult for sperm to penetrate), and possibly reduce tubal transport of both the sperm and the egg in their appropriate directions.

In women who are of no more than average weight, *Norplant* is 99.0 to 99.8 percent effective in the first year and 96.5 to 98.9 percent effective over five years. These rates are less for obese women.

Like all progestin-only birth control modalities, *Norplant* has been associated with irregular bleeding in more than 80 percent of users. This bleeding may be only staining or it may be more like menstrual flow. It usually subsides within the first few months but may last up to one year. Other side effects include mild bloating, headache, and breast tenderness. These and other mild premenstrual-like symptoms usually resolve over time. The rods of the device are not uncomfortable, but some women find them aesthetically unacceptable.

There are some disadvantages associated with the insertion of the device. It requires a surgical procedure before the end of the first week of a woman's cycle. The procedure is performed using local anesthesia, and some women report slight pain at the insertion site or pain or itching soon after insertion. However, infection at the site has been reported in less than 1 percent of cases. Spontaneous expulsion of the rods can also occur, but this usually tends to happen within the first month after insertion.

Norplant can be removed at any time within five years of insertion if you want to change birth control methods or want to become pregnant. However, removal of the device also requires another surgical procedure and sometimes involves tedious retrieval of the rods, which can be embedded in the tissue under the skin.

Norplant offers the advantages of onetime insertion and continuous birth control for five years. By reducing and finally stopping menstrual flow, *Norplant* reduces the incidence of anemia with long-term use. As a progestin-only device, it causes no estrogen-related complications (blood clots, cardiovascular problems, migraines).

One of *Norplant*'s greatest disadvantages, however, is its initial cost. The price of the device plus the office visit and surgical insertion varies widely, but it averages between $500 and $900. This total amount is required in full at the time of insertion. Removal fees run between $150 and $250. Over five years this cost is not enormously unreasonable; however, if you are not happy with the device or wish to become pregnant and want early removal, the overall cost can prove to be quite high.

DMPA (*Depo-Provera*)

Long-acting, slow-releasing hormones delivered by injection or by implantable devices are being developed. There have been two injectable hormone preparations available for many years, and their use as contraceptives has been controversial. In mid-1992, one of these injectable agents was approved by the FDA for birth control use. Depomedroxy progesterone acetate (DMPA, or the brand name *Depo-Provera*) is the only injectable progesterone available in the United States. One study had linked a higher risk of breast cancer in beagles that were given DMPA, but widespread use of DMPA as a human contraceptive in almost 100 countries has not borne out this risk.

The all-progestin, long-acting injectables act in much the same way as progestin-only birth control pills and *Norplant*. The pregnancy rate associated with DMPA is less than 6 percent. Progesterone works by reducing both ovulation and the motility of cells lining the fallopian tube by thinning the uterine lining and making the cervical mucus less penetrable by sperm. These effects last for almost four months, so to prevent pregnancy, repeat injections of DMPA should be administered every 90 days. If you do wish to become pregnant, you should not expect to regain fertility until four to twelve months after your last injection.

Like other progestin-only birth control methods, DMPA is associated with irregular bleeding for up to one year or longer. However, more than half of the women who use this form of birth control experience total loss of bleeding within a year. Other side effects common to progesterone-containing products include headaches, bloating, breast tenderness, and modest weight gain. An increased risk of cardiovascular problems, such as blood clots or heart attack, has not been shown to be associated with DMPA. To date, there have been no reliable studies to indicate the long-term effects of DMPA on blood lipids (cholesterol, LDL, VLDL, and HDL). Because DMPA reduces or stops monthly uterine blood loss, it can be a very important birth control option for women who have bleeding disorders or who are prone to anemia. There is also some indication that DMPA reduces the risk of developing cancer of the uterine lining and perhaps ovarian cancer as well.

Some other hormonal injection formulations are being studied. These contain estrogen and may prove effective in reducing the irregular bleeding. If irregular bleeding could be minimized, then the most common reason for discontinuing progestin-only injections would be eliminated.

The cost to the patient for an injection of DMPA is about $45. It should again be noted that it may take up to a year to regain fertility after discontinuing Depo-Provera.

The Intrauterine Device (IUD)

Intrauterine devices (IUDs) are a highly effective means of birth control that are widely available all over the world. IUDs are small plastic devices wrapped with copper and sometimes infused with progesterone. They are inserted into the uterine cavity and inhibit pregnancy. The actual mechanism of how they work is not entirely understood. They are thought to prevent the implantation of the fertilized egg in the uterine lining by creating chronic uterine irritation that is inhospitable to the egg. In addition, they seem to exert a toxic effect on sperm while also reducing the ability of the egg to be fertilized.

IUDs were widely available in the 1970s. Unfortunately, one brand available at the time, the Dalkon Shield, was associated with a high rate of pelvic infections that sometimes led to infertility. In fact, it was not the Dalkon Shield itself that caused the pelvic infections, but rather the polyfilament string protruding from the end of the Dalkon Shield. The string facilitated the transport of infective organisms (bacteria, including chlamydia and mycoplasma) into the uterus. Other, safer IUDs with monofilament strings have since been developed, but media attention to the Dalkon Shield made many women fearful of IUDs in general.

In the mid-1980s, all brands of IUDs but one were removed from the U.S. market. This was done not because all were unsafe, but in response to the epidemic of lawsuits that spread to IUD manufacturers, making future production unprofitable and product liability insurance impossible to obtain. In other parts of the world, however, the IUD remains an inexpensive birth control option for those women who chose to use it.

Although two types of IUDs are again available to women in the United States, many women remain fearful of them and will not consider them when evaluating their birth control options. Like all other forms of birth control, the IUD has risks and benefits; it is not right for every woman. But its renewed availability does allow women to evaluate whether the IUD would be a good contraceptive choice.

An IUD should be inserted during a menstrual period. This is done for two reasons. During a woman's period, the cervix is slightly open, making the cramping associated with insertion less severe. Also, there is little chance that a woman would be pregnant at that time. Before IUD insertion, a thorough pelvic exam and Pap smear should be performed and the results should be normal. Cultures of the cervix and vagina should also be obtained and treated appropriately. Inserting an IUD through the cervix in the presence of infection is obviously ill-advised; therefore, negative cervical cultures are very important. Some practitioners recommend that women take the antibiotic doxycycline—one dose in the morning prior to insertion and one dose in the evening following insertion—to reduce the risk of infection associated with IUD insertion.

The risk of uterine infection, which can spread to the fallopian tubes and ovaries, is still an issue with all IUDs. However, the risk for currently available IUDs is less than one-quarter of the risk associated with the Dalkon Shield. Infection associated with an IUD is highest at the time of insertion; therefore an IUD left in place for many years is least likely to cause infection. Removal and reinsertion of an IUD will increase the chances for the development of a pelvic infection. The IUD is an excellent choice of birth control for women who believe they want no more children or for women who want to put off future childbearing for many years. The possibility of infection may be higher in women who have multiple sexual partners. Consequently, IUDs are not recommended for them. IUDs are also not advisable for women who have had a history of pelvic inflammatory disease (PID). This refers specifically to an infection of the uterus, fallopian tubes, and ovaries, and not merely to the vaginal infections that commonly afflict most women at some time in their lives. If a pelvic infection does occur with an IUD in place, the IUD should be removed at once and an antibiotic should be started immediately. Infertility can result when the infection is left untreated or when it does not produce symptoms and silently progresses, involving the tubes and even the ovaries.

If pregnancy occurs with the IUD in place, the device should be removed at once. Sometimes this cannot be accomplished because the growing uterus will have pulled the string up through the cervix, where it cannot be retrieved. If the IUD cannot be removed, there is a 50 percent rate of miscarriage. That rate drops dramatically once the IUD is taken out. In addition, the IUD offers only moderate protection from pregnancies that implant in the fallopian tube or any other site besides the intrauterine cavity (an ectopic pregnancy). For this reason as well, IUD users who become pregnant should seek immediate medical care.

The two types of IUDs currently available are the "Progestasert" which must be changed yearly and the "Paraguard" which may be left in place for ten years.

The cost of the IUD in most parts of the world is very reasonable (about $40 in England, for instance). But women in this country must pay for the device as well as for the liability insurance and legal costs incurred by IUD manufacturers in the United States. As with Norplant, the IUD also has high initial costs associated with it. These include the initial evaluation, Pap smear, and cervical cultures as well as the cost of the device. The total cost varies from $125 for the "Progestasert" and $400 for the "Paraguard."

Sterilization

Voluntary permanent sterilization is the most common contraceptive choice made by couples in the United States. Sterilization procedures are indeed permanent and should not be undertaken unless a concrete decision has been made that no future pregnancies are desired. In neither males nor females are the tubes "tied." Rather, they are cut, burned, clipped, or in some way partially destroyed. It is true that operations have been devised for both men and women to reverse a sterilization procedure, but these operations are major, difficult, and usually unsuccessful. Because sterilization precludes future childbearing, deep and thoughtful discussions between partners and between couples and their caregivers should take place. The decision about which partner will undergo sterilization should be based on the risks of surgical complications as well as the psychological ramifications.

Vasectomy. The male sterilization procedure is called a vasectomy because it involves the removal of a segment of each of the two vas deferens, the channels that transport sperm from the testicles to the penis. The vas deferens is reached and severed through small incisions in the right and left sides of the scrotal sac. This procedure is performed in an office under local anesthesia. Sperm counts are then checked after 30 ejaculations following the procedure to ensure that the sperm reservoir has been used up and that no new sperm are present in the ejaculate. The vasectomy is the most effective form of birth control, having an efficacy rate of 99.8 to 99.9 percent. Complications from the procedure are rare and minor, and the most common include skin infections or temporary small black-and-blue marks at the site of the scrotal incisions. Certain recent studies have linked a higher incidence of prostate cancer with vasectomy, but they have not been substantiated. Male sexuality is not affected by the procedure. The ejaculate is somewhat less and thinner due to the absence of sperm.

Vasectomy is a relatively inexpensive procedure. The cost averages around $500.

Tubal ligation. Female sterilization procedures are called bilateral tubal ligation because they involve burning or removing a piece of both the right and left fallopian tubes. Access to the tubes is obtained either by opening up the abdomen with a 1½-to-2-inch incision usually made at the top of the pubic hair line or by inserting a laparoscope into a ½-inch incision under the navel. Both of these procedures almost always require and are best performed under regional (spinal or epidural) or general anesthesia. Once the tubes are identified, a small piece of the midportion is grasped and either tied and cut (when the abdomen is opened) or burned or crushed with a ring or clip (through the laparoscope).

The abdominal procedure is done in women who have medical complications that preclude the use of the laparoscope or in those who have had a vaginal delivery within the previous 24 hours. Because the abdomen is opened, there is a somewhat longer recuperation time involved and an overnight stay in the hospital after the procedure is usually required.

The laparoscopic procedure is usually performed in a one-day surgical unit, and the patient is discharged immediately after the procedure. Postoperative recuperation time is generally two to five days. This procedure requires a subumbilical incision for the laparoscope as well as a ¼-inch incision in the pubic hair line through which the instruments to burn or clip the tube are passed. Complications from this procedure can be minor, such as infection in, or temporary black-and-blue marks around, the incision sites. Other complications are severe, such as accidentally burning the intestines or injuring a major blood vessel. Major complications are rare (less than 1.7 percent of all procedures) but real. Depending on whether the tubes are cut, clipped, or burned, the efficacy rate is 99.1 to 99.7 percent. There are no long-term complications associated with tubal ligation. PMS and menstrual cramps are not made worse by tubal ligation. Sexual response is not diminished; if anything, it is increased once the fear of unwanted pregnancy has been removed.

Tubal ligation must be performed in a hospital or surgical center (average fee $1,000); it requires a skilled anesthesiologist (average fee $500 to $850) and a skilled surgeon (average fee for either mini-laparotomy or for laparoscopy is $1,500 to $2,500).

New Methods of Contraception

There are several new implantable contraceptives that are currently in the research stage. Two of these products are biodegradable, meaning that once they are inserted, they dissolve in a predictable way over time and do not require subsequent removal. Several new vehicles for delivering hormonal contraception are also being studied at this time. These include a patch containing estrogen and progesterone that is changed weekly for three weeks and then removed for one week. Another hormone-delivery device under study and further along in its research is the vaginal ring. This ring contains either a combined hormonal or progestin-only formulation. The ring is placed toward the top of the vagina during the first week of the menstrual cycle, where it slowly releases ovulation-inhibiting hormones. The combined estrogen/progestin ring is removed after three weeks and is replaced by a new one a week later. Each progestin-containing ring may be used for up to six months. A vaginal ring is not advised for women with recurrent vaginal, cervical, or bladder infections; for women with dropped bladders or uteri; for women who have difficulty holding their urine while coughing or sneezing; and for women who tend to strain with their bowel movements. These women may experience increased vaginal irritation and possible expulsion of the device.

Male Contraception

There are a few areas of male contraceptive research being explored in the United States, and some are being pursued even more extensively in other countries, such as China.

Male hormonal contraceptives are based on testosterone derivatives that work by suppressing the release of pituitary hormones that stimulate the testicles. That reduces the testicular production of both testosterone and sperm. Thus far, the long-term reversibility of injectable testosterone derivatives has not been ensured, and its overall effects on blood lipids have not been determined.

Gossypol, a natural chemical found in cottonseed oil, has been found to interfere with sperm maturation. It is taken in pill form first as a daily medication and then on a weekly basis. It has been shown to be more than 99 percent effective as a contraceptive; however, there are many side effects (such as decreased libido, dry mouth, upset stomach, fatigue), and there is a very high rate (up to 20 percent) of nonreversible sterility in men.

Surgically implanted silicone plugs have been tried both in women's fallopian tubes and in men's vasa deferentia. The success rate in women has not been high, but in men their use has proved more promising. In studies done in China, they seem to offer long-term, reversible contraception with few side effects. This "reversible vasectomy" has not yet been widely tested in the United States.

HOW TO CHOOSE A CONTRACEPTIVE

Contraceptive choice should be based not only on pregnancy rates but also on the convenience of use and general affordability of the product. The method of choice must fit comfortably within your sexual practices or you won't use it. Obviously, if you dislike or frequently forget to take oral medications, then the birth control pill is not for you. If you find a vaginal barrier method too messy to use or you just hate to insert it, then simply eliminate it as one of your contraceptive choices. If you are in a long-term monogamous relationship and you or your partner is tired of using condoms, then you (as a couple) have to reconsider your birth control choices. If you and your partner are not absolutely sure that you will never want one child, or more children, then sterilization should not be considered.

Teenagers should be able to discuss contraceptive choices with a health-care professional so that they can make a well-informed choice and protect themselves from unplanned pregnancies and STDs. They should be encouraged to be open with their parents but should not be denied access to information if they feel uncomfortable or unready to include their parents in these discussions. Condom use in addition to other contraceptive choices should be strongly encouraged to reduce the risk of STDs.

Women over 35 must weigh the risks and benefits of their contraceptive choice with the risk of pregnancy for each year past age 35. Because currently available oral contraceptives have lower hormonal doses than did those products cited in the very earliest studies, it is felt that the newer products are safe for nonsmoking women over 35. In fact, the FDA removed the "age restriction" warning labeling from oral contraceptive pills several years ago. A new ultra-low-dose oral contraceptive has been marketed for women who are approaching menopause. This new pill can be used to prevent conception and to control the irregular bleeding associated with the premenopausal years. Other contraceptive choices include barrier methods, long-term but reversible devices, and permanent sterilization.

For all sexually active couples, the contraceptive method they choose should enhance their sexual relationship by reducing the fear of unplanned pregnancy. A "good" choice is different for each couple and can change during the course of a relationship.

5

COMMON PHYSICAL PROBLEMS AND SOLUTIONS

With the health-care industry's recent efforts to inform the public of health risks, there has emerged a population of paranoid healthy people. Although educational campaigns should describe in detail which symptoms are dangerous and which are normal processes, this is frequently not the case. So much emphasis has been placed on instructions to call the doctor about any minor symptom that some people don't feel comfortable being more than a stone's throw away from their health-care provider. Many physical symptoms that women experience are actually very normal or benign, but such symptoms may be perceived as serious. This chapter will distinguish symptoms and complaints needing medical attention from harmless conditions that are within the range of normal health.

BLEEDING

It is frightening at any time to notice unexpected blood. For men it is always a signal that something is wrong, and investigation is warranted. But for women monthly bleeding is a way of life, and women learn very quickly what is a normal amount of bleeding for them. Some women bleed very heavily for a day or two of their menses, soaking as much as a pad or tampon every hour. For other women this would be a very scary event, because they might be used to three days of only very light flow. So even though bleeding is a monthly event for women, there are still times when they wonder whether it is normal.

Excess Bleeding During a Monthly Period

Most often an extremely heavy period is nothing to worry about, aside from the inconvenience of it. If you are bleeding more heavily than you normally do, or if the bleeding lasts a few days longer than usual, the explanation is usually a simple one. If you are a teenager whose periods have not quite regulated yet, a heavy period occasionally is well within the normal range. If your periods have been light for years and suddenly you have an abnormally heavy one, it could be a cycle during which you failed to ovulate for one reason or another. This might be caused by a change in exercise habits or a drastic change in diet, or it might be caused by an emotional crisis. It may also be a fluke month in which you didn't release an egg, and your period is therefore heavier because of it. If the bleeding tapers off and stops within a seven- to eight-day period and returns to normal the following month, there is no need to make a frantic call to your doctor. Taking 800 milligrams of ibuprofen (four 200 mg tablets) every six hours will lighten the bleeding and relieve cramps. You should always take ibuprofen on a full stomach. Try to limit activity on the heaviest days, and don't make your life too miserable by wearing white pants or being miles from a bathroom. Always carry extra pads or tampons so that heavy bleeding won't catch you terribly unprepared. If you are ready for it, menstruation is less upsetting.

If you have been trying to conceive or have been having unprotected intercourse and experience a very heavy period, there is a chance that it could be a very early miscarriage. The fertilized egg implants in the uterus at about the time you would expect your next period. Sometimes spotting occurs, which is not dangerous. Sometimes the egg is fertilized but does not implant properly in the uterus, and heavy bleeding will pass the fertilized egg as well as the uterine lining. When all is passed, the bleeding will taper off and eventually stop. If you have been trying to conceive, a miscarriage can be very upsetting. However, there is not much that can be done about it from a medical standpoint. At this early stage the only option is to let nature take its course and continue trying to conceive. There is often no way to confirm this diagnosis, since pregnancy usually isn't confirmed until after a period is missed. There is no need to be seen by your healthcare provider in this instance. The bleeding tapers and stops on its own.

Bleeding Between Periods

If you are not taking birth control pills and experience some bleeding between your periods, some investigation is warranted. It is important for you to take note of the circumstances surrounding the bleeding and the frequency of occurrence. In midcycle, women may experience a sharp pain in one of their ovaries, followed by an episode of spotting. This can be scary when it happens, but if it is not associated with any other symptom, it is most probably due to ovulation and will resolve itself. Any symptoms related to ovulation should not last longer than a day.

If you are taking birth control pills, bleeding between periods (breakthrough bleeding) is merely a nuisance. It does not mean that anything is wrong. If you skipped your pill for a day or more, or even if you were late taking your pill, the chances are high that you will spot a bit. The hormonal content of current pills is the lowest dose possible to prevent pregnancy and also to prevent harmful side effects. This low dosage of hormones makes the balance a little more delicate, and it is therefore more important for you to take the pills at the same time every day to prevent bleeding. If bleeding occurs, you do not need to call your practitioner. Stay on your schedule of pill taking. If you missed a pill, take it as soon as you remember and take the next one on time. The bleeding should stop, and you should get your period at the appropriate time.

Some women will have breakthrough bleeding even though they have not missed any pills and have taken them faithfully at the same time every day. This is truly a nuisance, but nothing more. Don't panic. Continue taking your pills. See what happens over the next couple of months. It can take your body three months or so to get used to the pills. If after the fourth cycle you still have breakthrough bleeding, call your practitioner to see about changing brands. Some women react better to certain kinds than others, and changing brands is usually all that's required to solve this problem. It is helpful to wait four cycles even if the bleeding really bothers you, as your body will never quite adjust to any brand if you keep jumping around from pill to pill. If you know that the breakthrough bleeding is harmless and you feel good on the pill you are taking, you don't have to switch. Some women feel that as long as they know it's not harmful, they can live with it. It's a personal choice.

Women who have painless bleeding between periods that is not linked to any other symptoms should really be seen by a practitioner. If your health-care provider is a nurse-practitioner or midwife, she or he may need to consult with a physician in this case. This is especially true if you are over 40 years old. An in-depth history should be taken and a complete physical should be done, including a Pap smear and a check for infection. Your doctor may also want to do an endometrial biopsy to rule out cancer or precancerous changes in the cells that line the uterus.

Bleeding After Intercourse

Bleeding after sexual intercourse is more common during pregnancy, when the cervix is engorged with blood. Deep penetration by the penis may irritate the cervix, and some bleeding may result. This can be terribly frightening, because any bleeding during pregnancy makes one immediately think that the fetus is at risk. Don't panic. Calmly get a pad (not a tampon), put it between your legs, and try to relax. The bleeding should subside fairly quickly and should not soak more than one pad. If the bleeding stops within three hours and was not more than that of a light period, there is no need to do anything else. You don't really need to call your doctor or midwife for this amount of bleeding if it followed vigorous sex. Just be more gentle next time. You do need to call your practitioner if you soak more than a pad an hour or if the bleeding doesn't stop after three hours. In those instances it is more likely that the bleeding came from inside the uterus rather than from the cervix. It could be that the placenta is implanted close to the cervix or over the cervix, which is known as a placenta previa. Any jarring of the cervix with a placenta previa can cause massive bleeding and necessitate premature delivery by cesarean section. If the placenta is over the cervix, you will have to abstain from intercourse. (Forms of sexual play that do not involve vaginal penetration remain permissible.) If the placenta is close to, but not covering, the cervix in early pregnancy, it may be pulled up and away from the cervix as the uterus grows upward. By six months of pregnancy, ultrasound can confirm the location of the placenta. If the placenta doesn't move, you'll have to abstain from intercourse until after delivery. Placenta previa is a rare condition, and most of the time during pregnancy sexual intercourse is perfectly safe and pleasurable.

If bleeding occurs after intercourse and you are not pregnant, there can be several causes. A small polyp arising from inside the cervix may be protruding from the cervical opening. Polyps are small growths that are almost always benign and that bleed easily on contact, but they can easily be removed at the time of a pelvic exam. Any type of infection will irritate the cervix and make it friable (i.e., cause it to bleed easily with contact). When an infection is present, there may be bleeding after intercourse. This may be the only sign that there is an infection, so it's important to make an appointment to be seen by your practitioner. An exam should be done and cultures taken to identify what organism (if any) is the cause. If you have not had a Pap smear recently, one should be taken to ensure that the cervix is free of pre-cancerous lesions. When intercourse causes the bleeding, the cervix is usually the source.

Bleeding from the Rectum

The most common cause of bleeding from the rectum is hemorrhoids. Hemorrhoids are varicose veins in the anus and rectum that are en-gorged with blood, and they can bleed very easily. Hemorrhoids may be internal or external. If they are external, you usually know you've got them. They are painful and make bowel movements exceedingly unpleasant. Internal hemorrhoids may or may not produce symptoms.

Hemorrhoids in women are much more common during preg-nancy, when the weight of the fetus presses on all the major blood vessels. Women also tend to be more constipated during pregnancy, and this will increase the occurrence of hemorrhoids dramatically. A hard stool will often cause some bleeding when you've got hemor-rhoids. Diarrhea will do the same thing. This is especially true if the hemorrhoids become thrombosed, which means they contain a small blood clot. Thrombosed hemorrhoids are very painful and may need to be lanced surgically to remove the clot. This procedure—performed by a surgeon—is quick and simple, and provides instant relief. It usu-ally will resolve the bleeding as well. If the hemorrhoids are not the result of a temporary condition like pregnancy or constipation, but are a chronic problem, you may need to have them surgically removed. A high-fiber diet and plenty of water will help prevent constipation, which can lead to hemorrhoids.

Bleeding from the rectum that is not associated with hemorrhoids needs a medical workup. In fact, a test for blood in the stool should be part of a routine gynecological exam, especially for women over 40. Painless rectal bleeding can be a warning sign of cancer.

Bleeding with Anal Intercourse

Because anal sex easily tears the rectal mucosa, bleeding is common. That method should be stopped temporarily to give the tissues a chance to heal, or avoided entirely.

Bleeding with Urination

Whenever there is blood in the urine, a urinary tract infection (UTI) is suspected. Usually there is intense pain and burning while urinating. Antibiotic therapy should be started immediately; you should be drinking lots of fluids as well (see chapter 9). A UTI can be diagnosed by doing a simple laboratory analysis of the urine. If symptoms are severe, the cause may be obvious, the lab test waived, and treatment begun at once. If UTIs are recurrent, your health-care provider may have a urine culture done. This will enable the provider to choose a more appropriate antibiotic to treat your infection. If urinary tract infection is not the cause of blood in the urine, a more thorough workup is warranted.

PAIN

Pain is usually a defense mechanism produced by our bodies to tell us when something is wrong. Pain in any form is a sign that some precaution needs to be taken. In a woman's lifetime, however, there are some times when pain is a normal process—mainly during reproduction. Labor and delivery are often the most painful events in a woman's life, and that is a natural, normal process. Cramps associated with menses are also a normal phenomenon as long as they do not interfere with the activities of daily living. Most women become accustomed to a certain amount of cramping before or during their menstrual periods. A mild over-the-counter pain reliever is usually all that is needed to relieve the cramps. Mild menstrual cramps may warrant your cutting back on strenuous physical activity, such as skiing or intense aerobic workouts. However, when a period becomes so painful that you cannot function as you usually do, a call to your health-care provider is warranted. You may need a prescription for a stronger pain reliever, or you may have a medical problem that requires some investigation. Endometriosis can cause very painful periods. A cyst on the ovary or one that has leaked or ruptured may be the cause of your pain. This cyst may resolve on its own, and when it does, the pain should not last more than a couple of days. If the pain lasts longer than that, it should be thoroughly investigated.

Painful Breasts

The ducts, glands, and lymph nodes in the breasts swell before your period and cause some tenderness. Your nipples may also become extremely sensitive for a few days before or after your period. These are normal occurrences and need no treatment. Some women find that a reduction in caffeine intake reduces premenstrual breast tenderness. A firm, supportive bra can help to alleviate some of the tenderness, because the breasts will not move or bounce as much with physical activity. A painful lump felt in the breast is most often a swollen breast gland. Cancerous lumps found in the breast are usually not painful. If you have a painful lump in one breast, check the same area on the other breast. If you feel a lump there, these lumps are usually nothing to worry about. Check again a few days after your period and they should be gone. If you have them throughout your cycle, however, make an appointment to have your health-care provider check them.

Pain with Urination

Urination should never be painful. If you experience a burning sensation when you pass urine, followed by a feeling of pressure, call your practitioner at once: You may have a urinary tract infection. If you have the burning sensation only when the urine touches your labia, you may have some infection or other process affecting the labial and vaginal tissue. You should seek medical advice for this situation.

Pain with Intercourse

Intercourse should never be painful, although there are many times when it is. If you are experiencing some pain during sex, a thorough investigation is needed to determine and alleviate the problem. This should be done as soon as the problem is recognized. If the pain is not severe, there are a few things you can do on your own. The most common cause of painful intercourse is vaginal dryness. This can be cyclical, occurring just after your menstrual period, especially if you've used superabsorbent tampons that not only absorb blood but also absorb normal vaginal lubricating discharge. It can also occur while breast-feeding, as you are estrogen-suppressed at this time and there-fore more likely to experience vaginal dryness. Menopausal women may also have this complaint, because they are also low on estrogen, the hormone that stimulates vaginal lubrication. If this is the case, spending a little extra time enjoying foreplay before intercourse will help to stimulate some vaginal lubrication. You can also use a water-based lubricant to ease the initial penetration. Saliva also works very well.

If the pain seems to involve more than just superficial tissue, if it occurs in the abdomen with penetration, or if the additional lubrica-tion doesn't help, you should be examined by your practitioner. You may be harboring an infection that needs treatment or have a growth or cyst that needs removal. Be sure to tell your practitioner that you are having pain during sex. He or she should always ask that question when obtaining a history, but if not, it is imperative that you offer this information.

Lower Abdominal Pain

Pain in the abdomen that is not associated with sex or the menstrual cycle also needs investigation. First, a clear-cut medical history is needed. Before talking with your practitioner, consider the answers to the following questions: How long have you had the pain? Are there any accompanying symptoms like fever or vomiting? Is the pain associ-ated with any bodily function like urination or defecation? When was your last bowel movement? Do you have the pain occasionally or all the time? Does the pain radiate anywhere, like up your back or down your legs? Have you been able to eat or drink during the pain? Does anyone else in the family have similar symptoms? Have you recently missed a period or had a positive pregnancy test?

Abdominal pain is a very general complaint and could mean anything from constipation to intestinal flu, acute appendicitis, or ectopic pregnancy. If the pain is severe, with a sudden onset, and is accompanied by a fever or vomiting, call your doctor right away. These symptoms usually accompany more serious diagnoses (like appendicitis and ectopic pregnancy), which require immediate attention. You should be seen immediately—in an emergency room if it is after office hours.

VAGINAL DISCHARGE

Normally, there is a discharge from the vagina, and it changes slightly depending on where you are in your cycle. The cycle begins with bloody discharge, which is your menses. Following this, there is a small amount of thickish discharge; it is either white or clear when it is in the vagina, but may turn yellow when exposed to air. Therefore, what you see on your underwear will be slightly yellow. Just before ovulation the discharge becomes thinner, clearer in color, and copious in amount. This discharge creates an optimum environment for conception and fertilization of an egg because it accommodates easier penetration and encourages advancement of the sperm into the uterus. This discharge should last a few days, throughout the time of ovulation. After ovulation the discharge becomes thicker again, and lessens in amount. This lasts until the menses starts again.

When you are aware of the normal cyclical changes in the vaginal discharge, you will be more likely to notice any abnormal changes. The normal vaginal discharge will not cause any other vaginal symptoms. Abnormal discharges are usually accompanied by one or more symptoms, such as itching, burning, or a foul odor. Color is one of the first things to note when you have a discharge that does not seem normal.

A thick, white discharge that has small curds in it may be the onset of a yeast infection. This type of discharge is usually accompanied by swelling of the labia, intense itching, and burning (for treatment, see the section on yeast infection at the beginning of chapter 9).

A greenish discharge that is slightly frothy is almost always a sign of infection. This discharge may or may not be accompanied by other symptoms, such as burning, foul odor, and painful intercourse. It should be evaluated by your health-care provider. A culture will need to be taken to identify the infectious organism so that the appropriate treatment can be prescribed.

A pink discharge usually means there is fresh blood in it and that a specific kind of irritation is causing some bleeding. This should also be cared for by your health-care provider. Most irritations, either vaginal or cervical, are caused by infection. A pink discharge that follows a Pap smear, however, is normal. The test may cause the cervix to bleed slightly, and when the blood mixes with the normal vaginal mucus, it appears pink.

Brownish discharge is old blood. Sometimes the discharge at the very end of your menstrual cycle is typically a brown discharge. If you have had any bleeding during a pregnancy, the blood may continue to be discharged for several weeks off and on, and it will be brown in color.

Discharge from the Breasts

The only time that discharge from the nipples is normal is during pregnancy and lactation. The breasts may leak for several weeks or months after weaning a baby, and that is also normal. The discharge of colostrum (premilk protein) during pregnancy is either clear or slightly yellowish in color. Breast milk also appears clear with a bluish or yellowish hue. In rare instances, a woman may leak a tiny amount of breast milk or colostrum for a few years after breast-feeding. This discharge can be stimulated by very frequent breast self-exams or by frequent sexual stimulation of the breasts. Rarely this can occur in women who have never been pregnant. Any discharge from the breasts that is not associated with childbearing needs medical evaluation: The problem could range from a pituitary problem to breast cancer.

SWELLING

Swelling by itself is the body's usual response to injury. It is the body's way of immobilizing an injured area. For women, though, swelling may occur on a small scale in response to hormone production. The breasts often swell a day or two (and sometimes up to a week) before the menstrual cycle, sometimes increasing by as much as a full bra size. This is a normal cyclical change and should subside a few days after the bleeding starts. This swelling should always be bilateral—that is, one breast should not swell while the other doesn't.

A very common symptom of the premenstrual period is abdominal bloating. There are a few relief measures that may be employed, but they will not eliminate the bloating completely. A reduction in salt intake may help reduce premenstrual bloating, but this happens to coincide with a time of incredible craving for salt in many women. Modest swelling may also occur in the hands and feet before menses. This should not be so severe that shoes do not fit. If you can push your finger into your ankle and leave a mark, the swelling is greater than normal and should be evaluated by your practitioner.

ABNORMAL OR MISSED PERIODS

Abnormal periods are one of the most common gynecological complaints, happening to all women at some point in their reproductive lives. The word "abnormal" needs to be defined as something that is not normal to you, the individual woman. There is a range of "normal" when talking about menstruation that is defined as periods occurring every 28 to 30 days (but actually ranging from 24 to 35 days) and lasting about two to seven days on the average. This is the pattern experienced by most women. However, there are women who regularly have periods on a much different time schedule, and this could very well be "normal" for them. Once your periods have been established, which may take as long as five years after your first period, you should be comfortable with the pattern and recognize when something is out of the ordinary.

MISSED PERIOD

If you have been sexually active with a male partner, the very first thing that should pop into your mind after you have missed a period is the possibility of pregnancy. Even if you have been using a reliable birth control method, you need to consider the possibility of pregnancy.

The first step in evaluating the cause of a missed period is noting the type of birth control you have been using. If you have been using Depo-Provera or Norplant, missed periods are normal and to be expected. If you have been using a method other than the birth control pill, Depo-Provera, or Norplant, you should get a pregnancy test right away. The sooner you do so the better, because your future options for an unplanned pregnancy are more numerous earlier on.

If you have a negative pregnancy test but no period, some recent lifestyle changes may be the cause. Emotional stress can surely be the reason for a missed or abnormal period, as can a drastic change in diet or exercise. Crash diets and excessive exercise (working out for more than four hours daily or running more than 10 miles a day) can often lead to abnormal or missed periods.

If you are taking oral contraceptives and have missed a period, do not automatically assume you are pregnant. Missed periods are a frequent occurrence while on the Pill, and you should be well aware of the reasons for this if you are a Pill user. The Pill prevents the building up of the uterine lining every month, so there is less to slough off. This is the reason that your periods are much lighter when taking the Pill. Occasionally, there is so little buildup of the uterine lining that there is nothing to slough off, and a period does not occur. If you have taken your birth control pills reliably, meaning you have not missed any pills, there is very little chance you could be pregnant, and you should continue to take your pills regularly. If this is a concern to you, get a pregnancy test to ease your mind. Your anxiety can be put to rest quickly and fairly inexpensively.

If you have missed any pills during the month and have also missed your period, you should definitely have a pregnancy test before resuming your next cycle of pills. With a missed pill or two, the chance of ovulation increases, and it is prudent to be sure that you are not pregnant before you take any additional pills. If you are pregnant, the embryo will be exposed to the hormones in the Pill.

If you are not sexually active with a male partner and begin having abnormal periods, changes in lifestyle are the first thing to look at. Again, emotional stress is often the cause. If that is absent, any major changes in diet or exercise should be examined. You should also look at things like smoking cessation, alcohol or drug intake, or major travel. If you have no accompanying symptoms, such as pain, headaches, blurred vision, or breast discharge, it is very reasonable to simply wait it out for two or three months. In most cases your periods will resume normally. If you do have any of the above symptoms in addition to missing your period, you should contact your health-care provider for further investigation. There may be an underlying medical problem that needs attention.

6

$\mathscr{P}$SYCHOLOGICAL AND EMOTIONAL ISSUES

$\mathscr{I}$t is sometimes hard to separate sexual issues into emotional and physical types. Sexual arousal is obviously not based solely on cyclical hormone levels and physical technique but also on emotional well-being. Women who enjoy sex are most often women who feel good about themselves, who feel safe and loved in their relationships, and who are able to communicate their needs and desires to their partners.

Cyclical changes in your emotions are normal throughout your monthly cycle, and throughout your life. There are times, however, when hormones can affect your emotions more dramatically than at other times. The most notable times are prior to menstruation, during pregnancy, in the postpartum period, and during the menopausal and post-menopausal periods. During these times, each woman's individual experience of sexual enjoyment may be very different.

For example, for some women, sex can be more enjoyable during the premenstrual period because they feel more sexually aroused during this part of their cycle. However, for other women, the premenstrual period is one of minimal sexual desire. For those women who experience breast hypersensitivity, premenstrual sexual fondling may be painful or repulsive. For women who experience cramps before or during their periods, sex is usually not enjoyable at those times. All of these scenarios are well within the normal range. It is perfectly fine to feel more inclined to have sex during one part of the month than another so long as you accept that as normal and don't perceive it as a problem.

During pregnancy, sexual interest can vary from month to month. Also, different women have different sexual drives at this time. Although some women feel liberated by their freedom from using birth control, others become so anxious about the outcome of their pregnancy that they cannot relax enough to enjoy sex. During the later stages of pregnancy, some women feel too bulky and encumbered to enjoy sex; others find that the uterine contractions engendered by orgasm are both worrisome and uncomfortable.

Some postmenopausal women feel increased sexual pleasure now that the worries of unplanned pregnancy and contraception are no longer issues for them. However, a larger group of older women find that their sexual lives are diminished by a host of physical and emotional issues. These include illness, vaginal dryness, a change in weight distribution that may be disturbing to them or their partners, or illness or death of their sexual partners.

Many unresolved conflicts from childhood or painful past experiences can manifest themselves in ways that affect emotional well-being. If your emotions are interfering with your life, if sex is unenjoyable because of them, or if your relationships with friends, family, and partner are suffering, then you need to look at the possibility that a deeper problem exists.

DEALING WITH SEXUAL PROBLEMS

If you feel you have a sexual problem or conflict, you should choose a health-care provider with whom you feel totally confortable. An evaluation should begin with a thorough medical, social, and family history. Was or is there any chemical, physical, or sexual abuse in your home life? Have you ever had an uninvited sexual experience or one that made you feel uneasy, ashamed, or victimized? When you look back on your childhood and adolescence, do you remember those times as positive or negative experiences? Was your family structure so controlling that you didn't feel room for self-expression? Were you made to feel ashamed of your body or your body's functions? Was the naked body considered something shameful? Any of these issues could affect your current sex life.

Many problems have an impact on sexual desire and sexual satisfaction. There can be differences in a woman's sexual response (or lack of it) depending on whether she is with a partner and, if she is, how responsive that partner is to her needs. The issues that can affect her sexual desire and responses are classified by physicians into three clinical groupings. The first of these are called inability dysfunctions and they include a fear of sex, a lack of desire for sex, and difficulty or inability to become aroused. Unfortunately, the term *inability dysfunction* seems to connote that something is wrong. If you do have a lack of sexual desire but do not perceive it as a problem, it is not a dysfunction. If you have a partner, and infrequent sex is not an issue in your relationship, then it is not a dysfunction. Lack of sex or lack of desire for sex is a problem only if you have a partner who demands or wants sex more often.

The second group of clinical issues involves orgasmic dysfunctions, both "primary" (never having reached an orgasm) and "secondary" (having once been able to reach an orgasm but being unable to do so now).

The third clinical group is called intromission problems and includes vaginismus (an inability of the pelvic muscles to relax during sexual stimulation, thereby preventing penetration) and dyspareunia (genital pain caused by sexual activity).

The causes for these problems are manifold. Fear of sex may be related to childhood experiences such as sexual abuse, incest, or other troubling sexual experience. Or the fear may be related to certain religious training or parental and family influence. Sex may be associated with feelings of guilt or shame rather than reflecting healthy self-esteem. Or there may be an underlying physical problem.

Lack of Desire

Lack of desire for sex (low libido) is not uncommon in women, and the cause of this problem (if it is a problem) can range from poor body image to a history of sexual abuse.

Low libido may be associated with depression whether precipitated by emotional events (such as the loss of a parent or child), by a physical event (such as the diagnosis of a serious disease), or by a combination of both (such as a mastectomy). It may also reflect some emotional problems in a relationship; for example, sex may be unappealing if you are not getting along with your partner. If you find you are uninterested in sex, make sure you are not also uninterested in your partner. Boredom or dissatisfaction with your partner may be masking deeper feelings of anger or resentment. These emotional roadblocks require establishing new avenues of communication. If the two of you cannot create an open and nonthreatening means of communication, you may wish to seek professional counseling. If you find that your lack of interest in sex is coupled with uninterest in other life-affirming activities, you may be suffering from depression. Again, counseling and other psychological support measures may be indicated.

Lack of desire for sex may also be due to just plain fatigue. If you are overwhelmed by office work, housework, or caring for children or aging parents, sex may be the activity that seems least important and, therefore, least appealing.

Anorgasmia

Inability to reach an orgasm, or anorgasmia, may be related to many underlying emotional problems. Women who have been sexually abused, for example, often have great difficulty engaging in sexual activity, in becoming sexually aroused, or in allowing themselves to completely let go and enjoy the involuntary sexual response associated with orgasm. The revival of childhood memories of the shame felt at experiencing sexual arousal—despite the involuntary, compromising, and coercive nature of such a sexual experience—can later impede the ability of some women to move from sexual arousal to orgasmic release. Those abuse survivors who do finally allow themselves intimate contact and who enjoy sexually arousing activities often come to an emotional and physical standstill before reaching an orgasm.

Another basic problem underlying a woman's inability to reach orgasm is some difficulty in her current relationship. Many women who have trouble having an orgasm with a sexual partner have no trouble reaching an orgasm during masturbation. For these women, problems in reaching orgasm with a partner may be a matter of technique or difficulty communicating or understanding sexual desires. It's essential that couples be able to freely communicate exactly what they want. For those who are too inhibited to express their desires, some counseling may be very helpful. Some women think (subconsciously) that they don't deserve to be fulfilled and that they shouldn't expect it. One of the biggest causes of sexual problems is a troubled relationship. This then becomes a vicious circle. The less enjoyable sex is, the more the relationship suffers.

Inadequate arousal is another common cause of anorgasmia. The arousal phase in women is equivalent to the erection phase in men. Women may have many physical signs of arousal, including vaginal lubrication, increased tension in the vaginal muscles, increasing length and ballooning out of the upper two thirds of the vagina, engorgement of the labia and clitoris, increased breast sensitivity and nipple erection, and flushing of the skin. Although most women feel these changes to be important and sometimes dramatic, they are not as obvious as penile erection, so a woman's sexual arousal is not always apparent to her male partner. Your partner, whether male or female, must recognize and participate in generating enough sexual excitement to allow you to go on to reach an orgasm. If he or she tries to rush the excitement phase, then orgasm will be unlikely.

Problems of orgasm may result from sexual preconceptions that are unrealistic. Many partners expect that they will climax simultaneously during intercourse and feel that anything less is an orgasmic failure. The involuntary pelvic muscular contractions that characterize orgasm may be attained during vaginal penetration or from extragenital stimulation of any erotically sensitive part of the body. However, orgasm is much more likely to be triggered by clitoral stimulation. There are not two types of orgasm—vaginal and clitoral—but rather different ways to stimulate the physiological responses that lead to sexual climax. There is no prescribed way to climax, no right or wrong way. You should not feel ashamed or disappointed in the means by which you attain orgasmic release. In fact, the very idea of attaching value judgments to orgasmic response may inhibit that response altogether.

SEXUAL ISSUES FOR TEENS

Adolescence is a difficult period of development. It is the time when we separate from our parents, experiment with things that are new (especially those things that are enticing and forbidden), and develop our own self-identities. Teenage experimentation leads to many risk-taking behaviors, and with the physiological surge of sex hormones and the enormous peer pressure to become sexually active, sexual activity during adolescence has become more commonplace. Today, close to 85 percent of women become sexually active in their teens. Teenagers are bombarded with media and advertising images imbued with sexual innuendo. Nevertheless, many adolescents are denied sex education and the knowledge of how their bodies work. For many young women, lack of accurate information, rather frightening changes in body shape and functioning, social pressure to engage in sex, stresses in developing an identity, and gaining some control over life can lead to unhealthy sexual behavior.

Sexual promiscuity in adolescent girls often reflects low self-esteem. Teenagers with low self-esteem believe they do not deserve better than to seek sexual satisfaction without the emotional bonds and intimacy of a deep and loving relationship. This fear of intimacy may be related to many earlier emotional traumas. Girls who have experienced the love and loss of a parent through death or divorce can fear becoming too intimate in their relationships. Often they engage in multiple, superficial sexual contacts so that they are not vulnerable to losing yet another deeply loved person in their lives.

Young women who have survived childhood sexual abuse are often predisposed to problems of sexual intimacy. Inherent in childhood sexual abuse is a betrayal of trust, which later may not allow the adult woman to enjoy the emotional openness of an intimate, loving sexual relationship. Because these children received love and affection only in the form of sexual attention, they may later confuse sexual activity with emotional engagement and fulfillment. Abused children seek out love but in return receive coercive seduction and mistreatment. In adolescent life this victimization can manifest itself in many self-destructive behaviors, including drug and alcohol abuse, irresponsible sexual relationships, and suicide. Incest and other childhood sexual traumas have many ramifications in a woman's life as she matures sexually. Childhood abuse can lead to the avoidance of intimacy by choosing multiple sexual partners or by avoiding relationships altogether. Growing up with painful childhood experiences of loss or abuse does not necessarily lead to sexual problems, but any such experiences should be thoroughly explored.

Young girls may fear the sexual changes their bodies undergo during adolescence. In an effort to fight these changes and to gain some aspect of control over their bodies, some turn to aberrant eating practices. They either seek the severe food control and/or excessive exercise programs of anorexia nervosa or they choose the bingeing and purging common to bulimia. Both of these eating disorders are seen in adolescent girls who have low self-esteem, feel out of control, and reject the sexual urges brought on by the hormonal changes of puberty.

Anorexic girls become thinner and thinner but are never satisfied with their body image. They are initially encouraged by a society that equates thinness with beauty. As they lose more and more of the body fat that defines their female figure, they also stop producing female sexual hormones. These girls stop menstruating, thereby turning back the clock on their sexual maturation. By rejecting her impending womanhood, the anorexic girl can avoid dealing with issues of sexuality. Her only means of control is her iron-willed ability to undereat. The final, and sometimes fatal, stages of the disease are characterized by such excruciating thinness that the anorexic girl becomes physically ravaged and emotionally devastated.

Bulimic girls seek to gain control of their adolescent lives by overpowering their bodies' normal functioning. They choose endless cycles of bingeing and purging, gaining at least temporary security in their ability to create some sense of control. The binges and purges are usually secretive behaviors, and such girls often withdraw from social and emotional interactions. In this way they do not have to face their underlying fear of sex and the loss of control it may represent to them.

Sex education should be incorporated early into our teaching programs so that young girls can learn to be proud of themselves from an early age. Sex education should not be self-consciously singled out as a special entity but rather should be made part of the basic teaching of health and nutrition.

SEXUAL PROBLEMS DURING THE REPRODUCTIVE YEARS

A woman who feels good about herself should feel comfortable seeking sexual satisfaction with or without a partner. Experimentation with sexual self-stimulation might have been discouraged in some families. However, masturbation can be both sexually satisfying in and of itself and can allow for safe sexual experimentation that can then be shared with a sexual partner.

If you and your partner are having sexual problems (such as not enjoying sex or not agreeing on what is mutually satisfying), you should both take a close look at your relationship and ask some basic questions: How do you and your sexual partner now feel about your relationship? Is there open communication between you? Is sex mutually satisfying, or are you expected to perform solely to please your partner? Is there another person in either of your lives?

Problems in a relationship often lead to sexual problems, and difficulties involving sex may be the first hint that something else is wrong in the relationship. If you find that there are major disagreements between you and your partner revolving around the issue of sex (or another issue, such as money), look beyond it. What partners usually fight about are just smoke screens for underlying conflicts. More than likely, the real issues are power and communication. Know that you can resolve sexual issues (as well as others) if you improve communication and let go of the idea that if you're right, the other person must be wrong. If you have a good relationship and do care about each other's needs, you can find ways to meet those needs without necessarily seeking professional counseling.

You may, however, feel that you would benefit from counseling. It is always optimal when both parties see the benefit in it and agree to participate. Men are usually more reluctant to go than women, but if the relationship is truly in danger, even going with a reluctant partner is better than getting no professional help at all. If your partner is absolutely unwilling to go to counseling with you, you can seek individual help. Although this may suggest that the problem is yours and not a shared one, the first step in resolving a problem is recognizing that it exists. The therapist may be able to give you suggestions and some tools to help resolve the conflict, or help you come to the realization that this relationship isn't going to work if you are the only one willing to address the problems.

If you feel you have a problem because your partner wants sex more often than you do, some simple steps may be taken to resolve the problem. As long as the relationship is a healthy one, conflicts over sexual frequency can usually be cleared up without professional help. First, understand that this is a common problem between both heterosexual and lesbian partners. It is especially true for partners who are in long-term sexual relationships.

In heterosexual partnerships, men will sometimes want sex more often than women do. Men often use sex for comfort; they tend to want sex when they are upset in lieu of working out the anxiety-provoking issues. Women, on the other hand, have difficulty having sex when they feel this way, preferring to talk out the issues so that they may enjoy sex as a reflection of their peace of mind. Women tend to be more communicative than men and need that communication to have satisfying sex. Once this difference is recognized and understood, some compromise or plan can be developed that mutually satisfies the sexual needs of both partners. Lesbian couples may also have disagreements over determining what is a mutually satisfying sexual life. These issues are not based on gender differences but can be based on different hormone levels, varied work schedules, or deeper problems of communication and control.

When sex is a frightening event or you don't feel safe during sex, you may need professional help in resolving the difficulties, and your health-care provider should be able to refer you to a qualified therapist. Sexual anxiety may be triggered by memories of a bad sexual experience such as rape or incest; in addition, it may not be something you consciously remember. As more and more women are recognizing and discussing the sexual abuse they experienced, support groups are becoming available to help them sort out these frightening memories. Qualified therapists who specialize in this area can help women clarify whether their painful childhood memories actually stem from abusive experiences and can help to resolve these terrifying events so that women may go on to lead fulfilling lives.

MENOPAUSAL YEARS

We live in a society permeated by sexually charged symbols and messages, but one in which explicit and honest discussions of sexual issues are rare. This is especially true for older people, and older women in particular. When older men start a second family, they are often considered virile. When older women show sexual interest, they are often considered unseemly.

Aging is a process experienced by all of us. Since most humans have sexual desires, a thorough understanding of the aging process will serve to help us accept and respect our changing capabilities. Our physical and emotional maturation will surely change how we behave and respond to many facets of our lives, including our sexual lives. Sexual responsiveness, like all other aspects of life, will be different at age 75 than at age 25. If your expectations mature along with your capabilities, your experiences will not be measured as better or worse, just different.

As we age, the challenges to maintaining good health increase. Our bodies change shape and no longer conform to the firm, thin, wrinkle-free model thrown at us by the media. We suffer through the loss of loved ones—our parents and their friends, our friends, and our partners. We must face medical illnesses that alter and limit our activities. Even without illness, aging inevitably makes us weaker and less able to perform activities we once considered simple. It is not uncommon for the elderly facing these losses to suffer from periodic depression. Maintaining sexual health is a part of maintaining physical and mental health. Interpersonal engagement, shared intimacy, and sexual activity help sustain the older person through these very real diminutions and losses.

For women, the first dramatic physical changes begin during perimenopause (those months or years of hormonal change that precede menopause) and continue into menopause itself (see chapter 11). With the physical changes associated with menopause, the sexual activity you previously looked forward to may become uncomfortable or burdensome. Although interest in what was previously sexually exciting may diminish, that does not mean that sexual activity must stop. If you engage in different and satisfying means of self-stimulation, you can continue sexual satisfaction with or without a partner. If you have a partner, teach him or her how to participate in these activities so that both of you may engage in sexually satisfying intimacy. Since the needs of both partners may be changing, experiment together. There is no reason why you cannot continue to enjoy mutually satisfying sex whether it includes intercourse or not.

Sexual health, even for older people, is both a reflection of and a path to maintaining a healthy self-image. What we consider sexually attractive has to do with self-respect and the ability to communicate physically and emotionally with another human being, not just with another body.

MEDICAL ILLNESS

Many medical illnesses will affect sexual response. They will require overcoming both the emotional trauma as well as the physical changes they may incur.

Hypertension

High blood pressure may produce few if any symptoms; however, most of the medications required to treat the condition will affect the sexual responses of both men and women. These drugs can reduce lubrication and orgasmic response in women, impede erection and ejaculation in men, and decrease libido in both sexes.

Cancer

Two of the most common fatal cancers in women are those affecting the breast and bowel. The treatment of these two diseases often requires major surgery, and the patient may suffer from an extremely altered body image. Mastectomy and colostomy are viewed as physical disfigurements by some women, and they require a long period of physical and psychological adjustment in order to feel comfortable with their sexuality.

Arthritis

Arthritis causes severe joint pain and stiffness, thereby limiting physical mobility and interfering with positions that were previously comfortable for sexual enjoyment.

Heart Disease

Heart attacks may instill fear in both partners that orgasm will induce a recurrence and even death.

Prostate Disease

Prostate disease and cancer in your male partner require treatments that may impair ejaculation and create impotence.

The list of medical conditions that directly affect sexual function in women and their partners is lengthy. The diminishment of sexual pleasure because of a medical condition may be a major issue for those involved. If your medical caregiver does not bring up the issue with you, you should bring it up. There are many support groups from which you can seek advice, information, and emotional support.

SEEKING THERAPY

If you find that your sex life is not fulfilling, then it is important for you to take the initiative to seek help. Depending on what problems surface, your provider may be able to help you or may refer you to a therapist, counselor, or support group that can. The type of counseling or therapy should be suited to the specific problem. Most counselors or therapists now specialize in certain areas, even though they have the same basic educational background. For instance, some therapists specialize in eating disorders, some in incest survivorship, some in marriage or couple's therapy, and some in chemical dependency problems. It is most helpful to have this knowledge before choosing a counselor or therapist.

Ideally, health-care providers should have some background on a therapist before making a referral, but often they don't. The more information you have about a counselor before you see him or her, the better, but if this isn't possible, ask the individual therapist or counselor when you call to make the appointment. Explain the problem you would like to work on and ask if the therapist has expertise in this area. You should feel comfortable that your needs are being met, and if that therapist cannot meet them, he or she should willingly refer you to someone who can.

So-called 12-step programs modeled after Alcoholics Anonymous are almost always available for people with drug and alcohol problems. Support groups for incest and sexual abuse survivors now exist in most parts of the country. There are also widespread support groups that meet various needs of women confronting medical problems. The American Cancer Society has a Reach to Recovery program for women with breast cancer. The United Ostomy Association sponsors support groups for people with colostomies and ileostomies. And there are many hospital-based support groups for people recovering from heart attacks and heart surgery. These groups will address issues that underlie your sexual problems, but you may also find that more specific sexual counseling is necessary.

Individual therapy may be indicated if you find that similar sexual problems have recurred even with a new partner. Individual therapy is also helpful prior to couple's therapy to clarify the issues that affect your sexual relationship. You also may want individual therapy if your partner refuses to go to couple's therapy.

Many experts in the field today see most sexual problems as a symptom of some deeper underlying issue. Therefore, current therapy tries to address those issues before moving on to treatments that solely address the act of physical sex. In the 1960s and 1970s, sex therapy that focused mainly on achieving intercourse and orgasm was more common and more available than it is today. That type of sexual therapy was based on the principles set forward by William Masters and Virginia Johnson more than 20 years ago. Their initial program, designed to treat heterosexual couples, did so in an intensive two-week course of daily therapy sessions for couples led by a therapist team that included a man and a woman. This gradually led to sessions in an outpatient setting, with one to three sessions per week and lasting several weeks to several months. The goal of therapy was to allow partners to abandon past sexual discomfort in their lives and become relaxed and open with each other, thereby enabling mutually satisfying sex to occur.

Masters and Johnson developed different sexual exercises that, after days of therapy, would lead to sexual intercourse. Before embarking on these exercises, the couple had to agree on certain preconditions. These included forswearing any other sexual liaisons; stopping all use of alcohol, sedatives, or other mind-altering drugs; abandoning any attempt at sexual intercourse until their therapists instructed them to do so; putting aside old angers and sources of disagreement; setting aside specific time to perform assigned sexual exercises; and, most important, agreeing to be open and honest in communicating with the partner about sexually stimulating or sexually unpleasant activities.

The exercises progressed from intimate touching to exploration of those areas of the body that were erogenous. The couple could then proceed to oral and manual stimulation of the breasts and then the genitals. The last steps of the program encouraged the couple to masturbate each other to orgasm. The final step of the program for heterosexual couples included vaginal penetration in different positions, later including thrusting to orgasm. The therapist decided the pace of the exercises and when the couple could comfortably proceed to the next step without re-creating anxieties.

These types of exercises done in the presence of a therapist are rare these days. Much information was gained from similar studies, though, and it is still the basis for the research of many sex therapists. Today, however, it is more typical for the issues to be discussed with the therapist. Exercises are explained, and the couples generally go to the privacy of their homes to practice. This technique is most successful in couples whose sex life has become limited or whose life situations have changed. It is also useful for those who do not have the vocabulary to successfully address these changes.

If you are seeking a referral to a sex therapist, consult your health provider, call your local women's health center, or find out if the medical center nearest you could recommend a counselor trained in the area of your specific problem. You (or your partner) must take the initiative to make the appointment. Also, therapy absolutely won't work if someone else is forcing you to go. Get several recommendations, and interview as many therapists as necessary to find the one with whom you can communicate. If you are committed to your relationship with your partner, then it deserves the work required to attain the mutual respect and dialogue that will lead to emotional and sexual health.

7

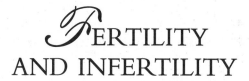

FERTILITY
AND INFERTILITY

FERTILITY

Most animals bear their young in the springtime so they can grow strong and survive the harsh winter elements, but human beings differ from most mammals in the timing of reproduction. Women have fertile periods each month, and therefore can bear children year-round. Males have no cyclical changes and are fertile all the time. When a couple decides to have a child, the process is relatively simple. Having sexual intercourse three or four times a week without the use of birth control methods will usually produce a pregnancy. In most cases, there is no need for detailed calculations or regimented sex. The majority of the time, sexual relations can be a spontaneous and loving process.

The monthly egg production in females is a complex hormonal process that is described in detail in chapter 1. Once the egg is produced, the fertilization process is a simple one. The egg is released from the ovary and starts its journey down the fallopian tube to the uterus. During the three days it takes to reach the uterus, the egg has the possibility of being fertilized by sperm while still in the fallopian tube. This is accomplished quite easily through sexual intercourse, when semen is ejaculated from the penis. As long as the male partner has no medical problems that affect sperm production and motility and has not had a vasectomy, the semen always contains sperm, usually in vast numbers. When the semen enters the vagina, the sperm move quickly through the cervix, through the uterus, and into the fallopian tubes. They can be in the fallopian tubes within seconds, which is why douching after intercourse will not prevent pregnancy. Hundreds of sperm will surround and try to enter the egg, but only one will succeed. Fertilization usually takes place in the upper third of one fallopian tube.

Once the sperm fertilizes the egg, the sex of the child is determined. It is the sperm and not the egg that decides the sex of the child. Women have only X chromosomes; men have both X and Y chromosomes, but each sperm can carry only one or the other. So if an X sperm enters the egg, the baby will be a girl; if it is a Y that enters, it will be a boy.

The timing of intercourse does not have to coincide exactly with the production of the egg. Sperm live for at least 48 hours, so even if intercourse occurred before the egg was produced, the egg may be fertilized by a sperm that was introduced a day or two before. This is why having intercourse a few times a week will usually unite the egg and the sperm at some point.

Once fertilized, the egg multiplies from one cell to two, then from two cells to four, and so on until a ball of 48 cells is formed. This ball of cells is called a blastocyst, and it will enter the uterus and implant itself in the lush and enriched lining.

The implantation of the egg happens at about the time a woman would expect her next menstrual period. With fertilization and implantation, the uterine lining will not slough off, so there will be no menstrual period. Therefore, a missed period is the first sign that a woman is pregnant. Sometimes implantation may be accompanied by a very small amount of bleeding or staining. Some women (especially those who were not trying to become pregnant) confuse this for a light period and miscalculate the dates of the pregnancy. Since the due date is counted from the first day of a woman's last menstrual period, noting whether the period was a normal one is essential.

PREGNANCY TESTS

If the pregnancy was planned and your periods have been regular, missing a period is usually all you will need to confirm that you are pregnant. Most women do get a urine or blood test for the detection of pregnancy hormones, but by the time they do so, it only confirms what they already know. If you have always had irregular periods or frequently miss periods, a urine pregnancy test is a very accurate diagnostic tool. The procedure is very simple: You can either take a urine sample to a laboratory (which will do the test for you—for a fee, of course) or you can buy a home pregnancy test kit (which is cheaper and almost as accurate). Just follow the directions on the box. The urine pregnancy test will turn positive approximately 14 to 20 days after conception.

The blood pregnancy test requires that you go to the lab, have technicians draw a sample of your blood, and then run a more sophisticated test on it. This test is the most accurate and most expensive test for pregnancy. It will turn positive as early as 7 to 10 days after conception.

IF YOU ARE PREGNANT

It is usually not until a couple of weeks after your first missed period that you will start to feel some of the effects of the pregnancy. However, some women have symptoms right away, with the most notable being nausea and fatigue. If you have looked forward to becoming pregnant and it was a planned event, the onset of symptoms can be exciting at first. It makes the pregnancy seem very real to you. However, this euphoric feeling usually fades rather quickly, as fatigue and nausea on a continuing basis become very unpleasant. Knowing why this happens might help you to cope with these symptoms.

After conception, there is tremendous growth and development of the fetus. Within the first few weeks the nervous, respiratory, circulatory, and digestive systems are all developing rapidly. Limbs and facial features begin to form by the fifth week. This rapid growth takes enormous amounts of energy, which your body supplies. That's why most pregnant women feel extraordinarily exhausted in the first 12 weeks of pregnancy.

Don't let yourself get too hungry. In early pregnancy, hunger can manifest itself in the form of nausea. The hungrier you get, the more nauseated you become and the less you feel like eating.

During the first trimester of your pregnancy, it helps if you listen to what your body is saying to you. Rest and sleep more. It may be frustrating for you to sleep your evenings away, but knowing that fatigue is normal and temporary will be of some help. Give in to your cravings and pamper yourself. Many women feel that eating certain foods will help make them feel better. Listen to that; it's okay. If you think that pepperoni pizza will settle your stomach, go ahead and eat it. Remember, you are not sick. It's not like having the flu and being nauseated. You don't have to live on saltines and Jell-O.

There are some other changes you will notice in your body during early pregnancy. Most women initially feel some degree of bloating. This is usually accompanied by breast enlargement and some tingling around the nipples, the result of the increase in the hormones estrogen and progesterone. The tenderness will diminish as the pregnancy progresses, but the size of the breasts will continue to enlarge, usually by several bra sizes.

The rapidly enlarging uterus (which before pregnancy was the size of a small pear) will grow to about the size of a large grapefruit during the first three months. This puts some extra pressure on your bladder, which in turn will make you feel the need to urinate more frequently. This is a very common symptom and does not indicate a problem. In fact, the nausea, fatigue, and frequent urination are looked upon as signs of a healthy pregnancy.

Along with the physical changes in your body, you will also notice many emotional changes. Once you become pregnant, it may seem as if your hormones have gone awry and you have no control over your emotions. Increased levels of estrogen and progesterone have a multitude of effects on the body, and mood swings are one of them. Mood swings occur throughout the pregnancy and during the immediate postpartum period, but they seem a little more intense in the beginning.

This is also a time when you are coping with a big adjustment in lifestyle. It all takes some getting used to, especially if you were the type who had lots of energy for everything. Now, when you only want to sleep instead of going to the gym, pregnancy may be a source of frustration and a sense of a loss of freedom.

By about 12 weeks after conception (the third month), you will start to feel much better. The nausea will be nearly gone, and you will start to feel like you've got some energy again; this will make your mood a little cheerier. As you enter the second trimester (fourth, fifth, and sixth months), the fetus will have formed all of the major body systems and will begin to move around, although you won't be able to feel that for several more weeks.

This trimester is usually the most comfortable of the three. You are feeling well and aren't quite big enough yet to feel encumbered. This is the trimester when you will start to feel the fetus move (called quickening), usually around 18 to 20 weeks for a first baby and as early as 16 weeks for subsequent pregnancies. This is an exciting event and makes the baby seem much more real to you. You can *feel* the presence of life. By 16 weeks or so in a first pregnancy, you will begin to show and will need to make alterations in your wardrobe (this tends to happen even earlier with subsequent pregnancies). At this point you don't really need maternity clothes; usually just moving up a size or two will give you enough room. These same clothes can also be worn after the delivery, since it takes a while to get back to your normal size. It is best to be well aware of this fact ahead of time, as it is very demoralizing to be unable to fit into your old clothes right after the delivery.

Many women worry about weight gain. In a society where thinness is synonymous with beauty, gaining weight can be a depressing outcome. You must remember that in pregnancy it is normal and necessary to gain weight. You are nourishing and creating another human being, and this takes energy and calories. Each woman gains weight at a differing rate during her pregnancy, but the general guideline is five to eight pounds during the first trimester, and an additional pound a week after that. That would make the average weight gain of about 35 pounds. Many women gain more than that; some gain less. The total weight gain should not be less than 25 pounds and not much more than 45 pounds. If you don't gain at least 25 pounds, it may be an indication that you are not taking in enough calories to meet the demands of the baby and you. The fetus will take the nutrients first; then your body will use what is left over for your needs. So in order to avoid things like calcium depletion from bones and teeth, fatigue, and lethargy, you need to be eating a well-balanced diet with additional calcium, iron, folic acid, and vitamin C. Your health-care provider and you should go over your diet thoroughly. There are many books available about pregnancy that give a detailed description of nutritional needs as well as providing other useful information.

Entering your third trimester, you will notice your belly growing at a rapid rate. The fetus is entirely formed, and its body systems are maturing. The fetus is also quickly gaining weight with the addition of subcutaneous fat, which accounts for the growth of your abdomen. You will start to feel a little bit more encumbered by your girth. You can't walk quite as fast and might find yourself off-balance a bit. By the last 12 weeks many of the discomforts of pregnancy have presented themselves, and you may experience one or all of them. Very few women escape pregnancy without experiencing at least one of the following symptoms: backache, breast tenderness, constipation, contractions, faintness, fatigue, excessive gas, headaches, heartburn, hemorrhoids, insomnia, itchy skin, leg cramps, nasal stuffiness or bleeding, nausea, nightmares, numbness and tingling in the fingers or toes, perineal pressure (sensation of pressure in the vagina), perspiration, pubic pain, round ligament pain (short spasmlike pain in the groin associated with uterine growth), shortness of breath, skin pigmentation, sore gums, swelling, alterations in taste, urinary frequency, vaginal discharge, and varicose veins.

Reading this list may be unnerving, but be assured that these are all normal, albeit uncomfortable, aspects of pregnancy. There is a physiological basis for all of them, and most of them can be made tolerable with simple relief measures. Be sure to inform your doctor or midwife if you are experiencing any of these symptoms or any other symptom that you feel is unusual. He or she will be able to offer you advice and reassurance. A professional will also be able to differentiate between the nuisance discomforts and any serious symptoms that might indicate medical problems with the pregnancy.

By the last trimester of pregnancy, you should have established a comfortable, trusting relationship with your health-care practitioner. Do not hesitate to note any symptom you are having and discuss it with her or him at your next visit. If you are feeling anxious about anything in particular, you should not wait for your appointment but call to talk about it as soon as possible. Such symptoms as severe pain or bleeding warrant a call immediately, even if they occur at 3 A.M. It is never a good idea to sit at home and fret over something. Usually a five-minute phone call is all it takes to ease your mind about the many strange feelings you'll have when you are pregnant. This is especially true if it's your first baby and you aren't quite sure what the normal symptoms should be. Keep this in mind when looking for a health-care provider for yourself during your pregnancy and birth. Choose someone you feel completely comfortable with and wouldn't hesitate to call if you have a question.

As the time for the delivery gets closer, you should be involved in some type of childbirth preparation, whether it is a formal class or an informal discussion with your doctor or midwife. Ideally, your partner should be involved in this, as partner participation greatly enhances the event and offers you a well-prepared support person. The changes of pregnancy encompass many aspects of your life and your lives as a couple. The bodily changes are merely one segment of a life-altering event that will forever change the world as you know it.

SEXUALITY IN PREGNANCY

Sex during pregnancy is a natural and normal activity. In the absence of medical complications, there is no reason whatsoever why you and your partner should abstain from sexual intercourse or other sexual activities. With the obvious physical changes you are experiencing, you may have concerns about certain aspects of sex. You should not hesitate to ask your doctor or midwife a specific question if you have one. Once your anxiety is alleviated, sex becomes much more enjoyable.

The most common concern of both partners during pregnancy is the fear that sex will hurt the fetus or possibly cause a miscarriage. Be assured that the fetus is very well protected. Nature has wrapped the growing fetus in a wondrous package made of a strong uterine muscle, amniotic fluid, and the mother's pelvic bones, which provide protection. Sexual intercourse, masturbation, and orgasm will not hurt the fetus.

Lack of interest in sex is another common complaint of pregnant women. Sex is usually the last thing on your mind during the first trimester, if you are nauseated and feel only the desire for sleep. During your second trimester, when you are feeling better, you may have a little more desire for sex. If you have no other children and privacy is not an issue, try making a date for sex. Set a time when you'll both drop what you are doing and head for the bedroom, maybe while dinner is cooking. Sometimes just changing your routine can be very helpful. Sexual desire erodes again toward the end of the pregnancy, when you are very large and uncomfortable. In addition, the movements of the fetus tend to be very distracting to some women, as if there were a third person to think about. The end of pregnancy is also a time when many women feel very unattractive and unsexy. It will help immensely if you can be open and honest with your partner and express your feelings. If the reason is that you're not feeling very attractive, express that honestly to your partner, and some reassurance that you are still desirable will hopefully be forthcoming. Everyone hates to beg for a compliment, but it could be that your partner is unaware of your feelings.

If the fetus moves a great deal, it may distract you from sex. If your partner is on top of you, a kick that hits you both tends to be much more distracting. Try some different positions that don't exaggerate the movements. Lie on your side or on all fours, with nothing against your abdomen. You'll still feel the fetus's movement, but it won't be as intense.

Pregnancy is a great time to experiment with different positions. The standard missionary position, with the partner on top, will be okay for a while. But as your abdomen grows, that position becomes uncomfortable at best and impossible for most. Be creative! Practice alternative positions and use lots of pillows in strategic places to add to your comfort. It's very difficult to enjoy sex if you are not comfortable. Putting some pillows under your buttocks will alleviate the pressure on your abdomen and will allow you to face your partner during sex, if that is a priority. Also, any position with your partner behind you, either with each of you on your side or with you on all fours, will eliminate the pressure on your abdomen. If your male partner is behind you, however, vaginal penetration is deeper, so it is wise to go gently at first. Sitting astride your partner in a semisquat during sex allows you to have control, and it is great exercise for squatting in labor. Try to use that position a lot.

Although sexual intercourse is perfectly safe in pregnancy, there are a few conditions that warrant abstinence. As mentioned before in chapter 5, intercourse will be strictly forbidden when there is risk of bleeding, as with placenta previa. This is also true when there is a high risk of premature labor. In addition, if your bag of waters has broken, you should not engage in vaginal penetration until well after delivery. The vagina is not a sterile environment, and because it is designed so that bacteria flow down and out, the introduction of bacteria is usually not a problem. Nevertheless, anything introduced into the vagina introduces bacteria. The uterus itself *is* a sterile environment, and the bag of waters is a protective barrier for the fetus against infection. Once the water is broken (a normal event close to labor), that barrier is gone, and anything introduced into the vagina could cause a dangerous infection in mother and child. Therefore, nothing should be put into the vagina, including a finger, vibrator, douche, tampon, or penis, once the water has broken.

There are two practices that should be avoided even if your pregnancy is uncomplicated. One of these is anal intercourse, in which harmful bacteria from the rectum could be spread to the vagina, cervix, and urethra and cause infection. In addition, hemorrhoids are greatly aggravated by anal intercourse. Ordinarily, oral sex is fine during pregnancy; however, your partner should never, ever blow air into the vagina. This can cause a condition called an air embolus, in which the air travels through the bloodstream to the lungs. This is a very serious condition that could result in death of the mother and consequently of the baby.

Apart from this dire warning, sex in pregnancy should not be feared or abandoned. At any time, good communication leads to a more satisfying and enjoyable sex life, and this is especially true during pregnancy. You need to be honest with your partner about your desire (or lack thereof) for sex, and you can be more vocal about what feels good and what doesn't. If those needs go unspoken, resentment rises and sexual intimacy suffers. Bear in mind that during pregnancy you are liberated from the use of birth control and you can be more spontaneous. Looking at the positive aspects of pregnancy and sex will help keep sex a fulfilling part of your relationship.

INFERTILITY

Infertility is defined as the inability to achieve a pregnancy after one year of unprotected intercourse. For a woman, *primary infertility* means that there has been no past pregnancy; she has never conceived. *Secondary infertility* indicates that a woman has had a pregnancy in the past but is currently unable to conceive.

Infertility is one of the most devastating things that can happen to a couple. Many relationships do not survive the emotional and financial stress that this medical condition can place on them. It has become such a focus in the medical field that there are doctors who specialize only in that area of gynecology. Millions of dollars are spent each year on diagnosis and treatment of fertility problems.

Incidence

Current research shows that one couple in six in the United States today is infertile. There have been no reliable epidemiological studies to show whether infertility is more prevalent now or if it is just more commonly talked about today. Infertility is now more commonly perceived as a problem and is a growing field of medical research.

After a detailed medical history and diagnostic tests, the cause of infertility can be found in about 85 percent of cases. Approximately 40 percent of all cases will be due to female factors, and 35 to 40 percent will be linked to male factors. In 10 percent of cases, there are combined male and female factors. The remaining 15 percent of infertility cases remain unexplained. With medical follow-up, about 60 percent of infertile couples nationwide are able to achieve a pregnancy.

Male Infertility Factors

The male partner is the cause of infertility in about 40 percent of infertile couples, and male factors are much more common than most couples believe. Many couples seem to assume automatically that the woman is the one who has the problem. Therefore, it is critical that an infertility workup not begin until both partners are present and willing to participate equally in the resolution. The diagnosis of male infertility is made by getting a sperm count. The test is inexpensive, easy to obtain, and physically painless. It involves bringing a room-temperature semen sample in a sterile plastic cup to a laboratory, where it is examined under a microscope for living sperm. Alcohol, drugs, cigarettes, and many medical conditions can affect the male sperm count. This analysis should be obtained *before* any tests are performed on the woman.

Causes of Female Infertility

The causes of infertility are broken down into four major categories:

Anovulation.   Anovulation, which means that no egg is released from the ovary during the monthly menstrual cycle, affects approximately 40 percent of infertile women. There are many factors that relate to anovulation, and they can usually be determined by a thorough history of a woman's lifestyle and menstrual pattern. Any woman whose cycle is less than every 25 days, or more than every 35 days, is highly suspect of being anovulatory.

Tubal pathology.   Tubal pathology is the cause of infertility in about 30 percent of women afflicted with this problem. If the fallopian tubes are blocked in some way, they will not allow an egg released from the ovary to travel to the uterus. They will also mechanically prevent the sperm from coming into contact with the egg and thus fertilizing it. This condition is diagnosed by a test called a hysterosalpingogram (HSG), in which dye is flushed through the uterus and the fallopian tubes and examined under X ray (see page 109).

Cervical pathology.   Cervical pathology is rarer than the two previously listed causes, occurring in less than 10 percent of infertile women. The cervix can be a factor in female infertility by producing either inadequate mucus or mucus that is hostile to sperm. Sometimes the cervix is so damaged by scarring (from a previous surgical procedure, childbirth, or a prolonged infection, for example) that it does not allow sperm to pass through it. The cervical mucus is capable of killing the male sperm, thereby preventing fertilization. This condition is easily diagnosed by a postcoital test. The test itself involves taking a sample of cervical mucus after intercourse and examining it under the microscope. It is best performed within two hours after intercourse but may be performed up to 12 hours after intercourse. With normal cervical mucus there will be a large number of sperm swimming around. If the sperm are not moving, or are moving very slowly, it is a good indication that the woman's cervical mucus is the problem.

Luteal phase defect. The luteal phase of the menstrual cycle is the part of the cycle following ovulation. It is usually 14 days in length, regardless of the length of the menstrual cycle as a whole. This means that there are 14 days from the time the egg is released from the ovary until the time your period starts. During this time, additional progesterone is secreted from the ovary to prepare the uterine lining for implantation of the fertilized egg (see chapter 1). But there can be a flaw in this process—for instance, if the ovary does not produce enough progesterone, the egg may be fertilized but never implant in the uterus. This is not one of the frequent causes of infertility, and it occurs in less than 10 percent of infertile women.

Unknown Causes. In about 15 percent of infertility cases, no cause can be found, even after extensive workups. It has been speculated that psychological factors may be significant, but these claims have never been substantiated and serve only to reinforce a couple's sense of failure.

Recommended Plan

If a pregnancy does not occur, there needs to be an organized step-by-step review of the problem. Some of the more simple explanations can be identified before you begin an infertility workup. It is wise to make note of the following history, as it will give your health-care provider a very clear idea of how to proceed with treatment.

The first thing to look at is your menstrual cycle. Do you have regular periods? If you often miss your periods or have them very frequently or infrequently, it may be that you are not ovulating. This is a very significant detail when caring for an infertile couple, and should be clearly understood by your health-care provider. With routine gynecological care and yearly Pap smears, your practitioner should already be well aware of your menstrual pattern and identify it as a potential problem before you even try to conceive.

There are a couple of ways to ascertain whether or not you are ovulating. The most simple and inexpensive is taking your temperature every morning (before you get out of bed) for one cycle. There will be a sharp rise in your temperature just before you ovulate. There is a special thermometer for this purpose. The basal body temperature thermometer, as it is called, goes from only 96° to 100°F, but the numbers are spread out to make it easier to see small temperature changes. The midcycle temperature rise will, therefore, appear dramatic. However, it is not essential to have one of these thermometers to identify the rise. An oral thermometer can be used, although it will be a little harder to see small changes.

Your temperature will stay at the elevated point until your period starts. The charted temperature (printed chart cards are readily available from any women's health center) gives you a clear picture of when your fertile period occurs and will therefore allow you to time sexual intercourse accordingly. You should be having sex at least twice during the three to four days surrounding your rise in temperature. This is the time during which the egg is traveling down the fallopian tubes and the prime time for fertilization. Therefore, you should be having intercourse every 36 to 48 hours. Having sex more frequently may decrease your partner's sperm count, thereby decreasing your chance of conceiving. Your health-care provider should be able to give you some chart cards with clear instructions on how to use them.

Other symptoms that indicate you are ovulating include thinner, more copious vaginal discharge that is stretchy if put between two fingers; bloating; breast tenderness; and irritability before your periods. There is a space on the temperature chart to record these symptoms on the day you experience them. It's very helpful to fill in all your symptoms. Some practitioners who deal with infertile couples suggest keeping these records for three months or more before the rest of the workup is begun. However, one month of basal body temperatures and recorded symptoms should be adequate to give the practitioner an idea if the menstrual cycle is the problem. If you have regular monthly periods, are able to accurately record your temperatures daily for one month, and find that a clear pattern emerges, then you need not continue charting your temperatures. Waiting three months to follow up on a problem that is so very important can be emotionally draining. It is unfair to prolong the infertility workup unnecessarily.

There is another way to confirm ovulation, and that is with a commercial ovulation predictor kit. Like the pregnancy test kits, the ovulation kits work by detecting a shift in hormone production. The kits are easy to use and contain detailed instructions. They can be purchased at most drugstores for about $30.

Many experts stress that a couple should not consider themselves infertile until a year has passed. Indeed, many practitioners will not start a workup before that time. However, some circumstances make it appropriate to begin a workup sooner. When there is a known problem it is senseless to wait a full year to resolve it. For instance, if your practitioner is very familiar with you and knows your menstrual cycles are anovulatory, he or she should begin suitable intervention as early as two months after you've tried to conceive. If you are an older couple trying to conceive for the first time, it may make sense to start the workup after only six months. Fertility in all women begins to decline after age 30. Between ages 30 and 35, the decline is very minimal, but after age 35 the decline in fertility progresses more rapidly.

If the frequency of intercourse seems appropriate, your male partner has no problem with erection or ejaculation, and you have not conceived, then it is time to see your health-care provider with your temperature chart in hand. (The chart should cover a period of one month or more.) When you make the appointment to see your doctor, midwife, or nurse-practitioner, be sure to indicate that the appointment is being made to discuss infertility. Much more time should be allowed for the visit, since there are many procedures and feelings to be discussed and the discussion may become very emotional.

The Workup

Your first visit to your health-care provider for an infertility workup should be an interview and a general physical exam including a Pap smear. The interview portion of the visit is the most important aspect of the entire process, because most causes of infertility can be identified by getting an accurate and detailed history of the problem. For this reason, the visit should be allotted an hour or more; however, in a busy practice these visits are usually scheduled for a half hour. No one should have to feel rushed to blurt out one's medical and sexual history while coping with the intense emotions associated with the inability to conceive.

It is important that you accurately recall any health problems you have had in the past, especially those having to do with the reproductive system. Any history of sexually transmitted diseases, thyroid problems, abortions, or abdominal surgery should be related in as much detail as possible. Menstrual problems are also very significant. Symptoms such as severe pain before or during your periods should be thoroughly discussed. And be fully prepared to discuss your sexual activity, including any pain during intercourse, failure to achieve orgasm, or lack of desire.

For men, difficulties in achieving an erection or ejaculation are issues that will need to be addressed. These issues must be talked about openly and honestly with a health-care professional. If the man does not feel comfortable discussing this with a gynecologist, he should see a urologist or his own medical provider. In addition, the couple should be able to talk with each other. Any information you withhold from your caregiver can impede the evaluation process.

The caregiver should be professional and sensitive to your needs for privacy and emotional support. If you have already undergone tests for infertility, it is important to share that information and, if possible, provide the record of the tests. There should be no need to repeat tests already performed. However, there are some practitioners who insist on doing them again. Make sure that the caregiver offers a valid reason why he or she does not trust those test results. If you are uncomfortable with those reasons, be very frank and open about it. You deserve an explanation about why an uncomfortable test needs to be repeated when it places a physical and financial burden on you.

After the interview, a thorough physical exam should be performed (see chapter 3). This exam gives the practitioner a vast amount of information that can aid in the diagnostic process. Cervical scarring (caused by traumatic childbirth, abortion, or infection) can sometimes be seen with a speculum, and the presence of adhesions and ovarian cysts is sometimes revealed by a bimanual exam. All of these conditions can contribute to infertility.

Diagnostic tests.   There are five diagnostic tests to be performed, including a semen analysis, a hysterosalpingogram (HSG), a postcoital test, an endometrial biopsy, and laparoscopy. The timing of these tests (except for the semen analysis) will depend upon where you are in your menstrual cycle. If you have already accurately recorded at least one month of basal body temperatures, bring this chart with you to your first visit and the tests can be scheduled right away. Otherwise, the next month will be spent obtaining this temperature chart and the actual tests will be scheduled for the following month. The semen analysis should be done as soon as possible after the initial consultation. There is no point continuing an infertility workup that involves expensive and painful tests for you if your partner has no sperm or is unwilling to be tested.

The HSG is performed early in the follicular phase of the monthly cycle—after the menstrual flow has stopped, but before ovulation. Because this test involves an X ray, it is done before ovulation to avoid possibly exposing a fertilized egg to the radiation. The HSG diagnoses intrauterine and tubal pathology. Dye is injected into the uterus and should fill the uterine cavity and then travel through the fallopian tubes and spill out the ends near the ovaries. The process is watched under X ray and takes about two minutes. Oftentimes, fallopian tubes that were partially blocked by mild adhesions or endometriosis are opened by this flushing and will subsequently allow passage of an egg. In this case the diagnostic procedure will effect a cure for the infertility.

The postcoital test is done as close to ovulation as possible and should be done within 6 to 12 hours of intercourse. This involves an office visit and a speculum exam. The quality of the cervical mucus is determined, and then a microscopic examination is performed. Evidence of infection is looked for and an evaluation of the sperm is done. There should be at least five progressively motile sperm in every microscopic area seen under the high-powered lens.

The endometrial biopsy is done several days before you suspect you will get your period. Tissue is taken from inside the uterus by inserting a thin tube through the cervix during a speculum exam. The procedure is painful and may be done under local anesthesia. The specimen is then sent to a pathology laboratory. It is examined there and will confirm whether ovulation actually occurred, and if the progesterone production is adequate to sustain a pregnancy. There are some practitioners who feel they don't get enough useful information from this test to warrant its pain and expense, so they may defer it until several treatments have failed. However, it is still a standard test in the infertility workup.

Laparoscopy is the most expensive test and the most invasive. This procedure involves general anesthesia and a small abdominal incision under the navel. A special instrument known as a laparoscope is inserted into the abdominal cavity so that the abdominal and reproductive organs can be seen. This is done on an outpatient basis, but a woman will require a few days' recovery at home before returning to her normal routine. This test is usually deferred for three to four months, since it is an expensive operative procedure. If endometriosis (an overgrowth of the uterine lining) or adhesions are strongly suspected, the laparoscopy may be done sooner in the workup. During this procedure the surgeon may use a laser or cautery to remove endometrial tissue and/or adhesions if either are found.

All diagnostic tests except the semen analysis can be done in any order. They should be begun according to where you are in your menstrual cycle and, aside from the laparoscopy, should be completed within one or two months. The timing should depend on the particular couple and their schedules. If you are both busy and want to wait before having some of the tests done, that is certainly your prerogative. You may also feel that you cannot emotionally handle doing all these tests in one month. It should be emphasized, however, that they *can* be done within one month, and your caregiver should not drag everything out over a six-month period if you are feeling that time is wasting. Once the tests are done, a treatment plan can be outlined and you can have the sense that you are moving forward in resolving your fertility problems.

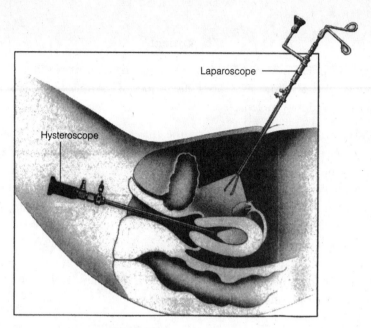

Figure 7.1. Laparoscopy (shown here concomitant hysteroscopy)

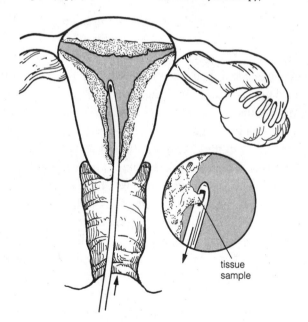

Figure 7.2. Endometrial Biopsy

Treatment

The treatment for infertility is obviously dependent on the likely causes. What follows is a brief discussion of various treatments for specific fertility problems.

Male Factors. If it is clear that the male partner has a low sperm count or difficulty with erection or ejaculation, he should be referred to a urologist (a physician who specializes in the urogenital tract). Sperm take three months to form, and they must be continuously replenished. Many environmental factors—stress, alcohol, marijuana, tobacco, chronic diseases, and environmental toxins like radiation—affect sperm production. For this reason, it is usually necessary to have more than one sperm count to ensure that the number and health of the sperm are consistent. If sperm are completely absent, the possibility of donor insemination can be considered.

Ovulation Disorders. If you are not ovulating, there are several medications that can stimulate the ovaries to produce one or more eggs. The most common medication is clomiphene (*Clomid*), which is taken orally on days 5 through 9 (or sometimes days 3 through 7) of the menstrual cycle. This means that the first pill is taken five days after you begin to bleed and then taken once daily for five consecutive days. The initial dose is usually 50 milligrams per day. If ovulation is not achieved during the first month, the dosage is increased the following month to 100 milligrams per day. The dosage is increased each month by 50 milligrams until the maximum dose of 250 milligrams per day is reached. The usual course is to keep taking the maximum dose necessary to achieve ovulation for four to five cycles before moving on to another medication. Clomid stimulates the ovaries to produce at least one egg, so it can somewhat increase the chance of producing twins. Most infertile couples are willing to take the risk of having twins.

Pergonal is another medication that stimulates egg production, but it is not taken orally. It can be absorbed only via injection. The incidence of multiple gestation is much higher with Pergonal because it hyperstimulates the ovaries, and many eggs may be produced. This is the medication that is known to cause triplets, quadruplets, and even quintuplets. There are obstetrical risks associated with carrying three or more babies, and these risks should be discussed with your practitioner.

Cervical Factors. If the cause of the infertility is poor or hostile cervical mucus, or cervical stenosis (narrowing), there are several therapies that can be employed. Taking low-dose estrogen orally or as a topical treatment before ovulation may improve the cervical mucus and enable the sperm to enter the uterus. It is thought that over-the-counter cough syrups (such as *Robitussin* and *SSKI*) taken before ovulation can also improve the quality of the cervical mucus because they tend to break up thick mucus. Intrauterine insemination, whereby a properly prepared sample of your partner's semen is introduced directly into your uterus, bypassing the cervical mucus, is also worth trying.

Intrauterine insemination is also recommended when there is a large amount of cervical stenosis that is preventing the passage of sperm. The procedure involves slightly dilating the cervix with a plastic catheter and injecting the semen through this catheter. This procedure is performed during a speculum exam, and may cause a small amount of cramping if the cervix is very tight and sensitive. There are rarely adverse physical side effects to this procedure, however.

Luteal Phase Defects. When the level of progesterone secreted by the ovaries is not sufficient to sustain the pregnancy (i.e., it will not allow the fertilized egg to implant), natural progesterone in the form of vaginal suppositories or micronized progesterone pills are indicated. The suppositories are inserted into the vagina twice a day, beginning just after ovulation and continuing until menses. The pills are taken by mouth twice a day. If this treatment does allow the fertilized egg to implant and pregnancy does occur, the suppositories or pills are continued at the same dosage until the first trimester of pregnancy is completed. The suppositories are more readily available, but they are messy. Once the suppository melts, it drains from the vagina. Thus, it may cause some swelling and breakdown of the skin of the labia, and urination may become painful. These symptoms are relieved with warm baths, but they will not disappear completely until the suppositories are stopped. The pills are newly available and are not as easy to obtain. They are much neater and easier to use, and they can be purchased through a centralized phone-order pharmacy.

Tubal Factors. If the fallopian tubes are severely traumatized or blocked, as can be found in severe endometriosis, scarring from infection, or past ectopic pregnancies, the treatment can take two courses. Microsurgery can be performed to repair damaged tubes (with no guarantee of success), or you can opt for in vitro fertilization (IVF). With IVF, the eggs are surgically retrieved via ultrasound and then fertilized in a laboratory with the sperm produced by the male partner. The fertilized eggs are then implanted into the uterus through the cervix.

These two options are very invasive procedures, and it is imperative that you discuss them at great length with your health-care provider and surgeon. Many gynecologists perform microsurgery, but in the case of IVF, the doctor must refer you to an infertility program at the nearest major medical center or specialized infertility center. Some of these programs have better success rates than others, with the national average being at least 15 percent. Some centers claim to have a 30 percent rate of success, and for a procedure as invasive, emotionally loaded, and expensive as IVF, it is very wise to carefully check out all your options. The average cost of IVF (one attempt) is $7,000 or more.

Because all of the tests and treatments rely on knowing where you are in your cycle, the basal body temperature charts must be done throughout the whole process. This can become quite stressful for a couple, because the infertility process is physically invasive as well as mentally frustrating. Regimented sex can lead to sexual dysfunction and increased tension in a relationship. In fact, the infertility process is so emotionally draining that many relationships do not survive it. The infertile couple is continually being offered another brass ring to reach for on the infertility merry-go-round. This is especially true in light of the many new technologies that are continually being developed. Just when you get to the point where you feel like stopping the process, a new hope is offered. Remember that this is your body. You as a couple are the ones to make the decisions about how far this process should go, at what pace, and at what cost. At some point the infertile couple must resolve how they define their family. This happens when the partners have their own biological child, adopt a child, or decide to live as a family without children.

8

ABORTION

Abortion is the medical term for the loss of a pregnancy prior to the twenty-fourth week, whether that loss is effected by natural causes or by outside intervention. Those pregnancies that terminate naturally are referred to as spontaneous abortions or miscarriages; those that are terminated by medical intervention are referred to as induced abortions or therapeutic abortions.

Miscarriage is an extremely common event. During the first 12 weeks of pregnancy (the first trimester), miscarriage occurs in 12.5 percent to 18 percent of all confirmed pregnancies. However, these figures probably represent a gross underestimation of early miscarriage. Newer information indicates that as many as 75 to 90 percent of all pregnancies are lost in the first trimester. The bulk of these miscarriages occur so early that the women never even knew they were pregnant; sometimes their period may have been a little heavier or a day or two later than expected, but in other cases there are no suspicious indications at all.

Why does miscarriage occur? When you consider the miracle of joining a sperm and egg to form a human being, it becomes easier to understand that many of these unions will not survive. Luckily, nature recognizes at an early stage most of the pregnancies that are not genetically viable and stops their continued development. Generally, the earlier a miscarriage occurs in a pregnancy, the less compatible with life the embryo would have been. In at least 50 to 60 percent of early miscarriages, there is some miscombination or abnormal amount of genetic material—either the wrong number of chromosomes or too many sets.

Sometimes the uterus has structural abnormalities (such as congenital abnormalities that were caused spontaneously or by dangerous drugs and other agents). In other cases, the uterus may not be receiving adequate hormonal stimulation, and the embryo will not have its proper lush bed in which to settle and grow.

There are other factors that may compromise the ability of the embryo to survive. These include viruses, bacteria, and other infective agents; high doses of radiation exposure; severe malnutrition; drug, cigarette, or alcohol abuse; and severe chronic disease in the pregnant mother. The degree to which the embryo or fetus is adversely affected by environmental substances and/or drugs is directly related to four factors: (1) the dose of the substance or drug, (2) the timing of the exposure of the embryo or fetus to the substance, (3) the duration of exposure, and (4) exposure to two or more substances or drugs simultaneously, allowing the two factors to interact and increase the potential danger to the embryo or fetus. Environmental factors, particularly if the exposure occurs in the first trimester, can indeed harm the embryo and even cause miscarriage. However, even extremely potent toxins are more likely to harm the embryo than cause it to abort.

In general, there are still a large number of miscarriages whose causes remain unknown, and most causes are totally outside our control. If you have a miscarriage, you may have feelings of guilt and assume that something you have done has caused it. These feelings are common, but they are completely unfounded. There is no strenuous activity you could do that would induce the miscarriage of a healthy fetus. Women who miscarry after shoveling show or mountain climbing have absolutely *not* caused the event: The timing is merely coincidental in those incidences. There are people who will try to provide you with reasons for the miscarriage (old wives' tales still run rampant on this subject). Most of them blame some undertaking that they are sure caused the loss of the fetus. These false assumptions include such far-ranging activities as lifting bags of groceries or the laundry basket to jogging or engaging in sports, wearing a seat belt, traveling by plane, eating particular foods, or engaging in sexual activity.

Despite all the "reasons" offered by others, it's clear that a healthy embryo and fetus are very strong, and that the ones that are miscarried are those not destined to survive. Although it may well be best that a nonviable pregnancy has not continued, it does not diminish the sense of loss and grief that occur at this time. Allow yourself the time and quiet necessary for you and your partner to grieve. When you have come to terms with what has happened, you can try to conceive again.

There are many terms that describe the different kinds of early spontaneous fetal loss. Light bleeding, or spotting, does not always signify that a miscarriage will occur. In fact, the pregnancy can go on to develop normally. In those instances, the bleeding may represent the very early loss of a second twin or it may represent transient bleeding from an unknown source, such as a low-lying placenta, or a small placental separation that spontaneously resolves. If bleeding does occur, an ultrasound can be performed to reveal what is taking place in the uterus. At a very early stage, you may see only the sac in which the embryo has started to grow. At a slightly later stage, you may see a healthy-looking embryo with the tiny flicker of the fetal heart. If there has been bleeding, the ultrasound technician may see an early, healthy-appearing embryo next to the collapsing sac of a twin that is being lost. In the case of a threatened abortion (bleeding of unknown cause without cervical dilation), the technician may see a sac that is beginning to collapse and/or an embryo that does not appear healthy. The technician may also see a normal viable fetus with no discernable cause for bleeding.

TYPES OF ABORTIONS

Inevitable Abortions

Inevitable abortions are characterized by spotting, or light bleeding. When the cervix is examined, however, it is found to be open in anticipation of the incipient loss of the pregnancy. If an ultrasound is performed, a collapsing sac and/or an unhealthy embryo may be seen.

Incomplete Abortions

Incomplete abortions are characterized by bleeding and the passage of some tissue. In such cases, the uterus is attempting to expel the unhealthy embryo and associated tissue. The bleeding is typically heavy and is accompanied by cramping. When the cervix is examined, it will be open and pregnancy-related tissue can usually be identified in the vagina or coming from the uterus. The ultrasound picture will either be similar to that seen in inevitable abortions or show only the thickened, lush uterine lining that remains after the embryo has been expelled.

Complete Abortions

Complete abortions are characterized by bleeding and cramping, and there will be a total expulsion of the embryo and surrounding pregnancy-related tissue. Upon examination the cervix may be partially open or may have already closed. The ultrasound will show a uterine cavity without any pregnancy-related tissue and with only the thin strip of the normal uterine lining present.

Missed Abortions

Missed abortions are characterized by a lack of expected growth in uterine size. They usually have no accompanying symptoms of bleeding, but many women do notice the loss of pregnancy symptoms such as nausea and breast tenderness. Often the diagnosis of missed abortion (also known as a blighted ovum) is discovered only on a routine obstetrical exam. Ultrasound confirmation of a blighted ovum reveals an empty sac with no embryo, or sometimes a sac with a poorly formed embryo. Many missed abortions would go on to bleed and become inevitable or incomplete abortions. But in medical communities where early ultrasound screening is available, this early pregnancy loss may be diagnosed before symptoms of bleeding or cramping occur.

If upon examination your health-care provider finds that you have partially miscarried, that you are about to miscarry, or that the ovum is blighted and will not develop, the recommended course of action is for the uterus to be emptied of its nonviable contents. The standard treatment of all but complete miscarriage requires that any remaining pregnancy-related tissue be removed from the uterus. If any tissue is left inside the uterus, it can provoke a serious infection. The procedure used to empty the uterus is called a D&C (dilation and curettage). It involves dilating the cervix, if it is not already open, and removing the remaining pregnancy-related tissue with either a suction or a sharp curette. The procedure is done quickly and is usually performed under anesthesia. Although you may have some bleeding after the D&C, the procedure will effectively stop any heavy bleeding and will also definitely end a nonviable pregnancy.

A miscarriage can be so emotionally traumatic that it's normal to be worried it will happen again. However, the chances that your next pregnancy will miscarry are no greater than they were the first time. Sometimes a miscarriage can happen twice in a row, but the success rate for a pregnancy following a miscarriage ranges between 70 and 90 percent. Repeated spontaneous miscarriages are more likely to be the result of chance than of any specific cause. Three consecutive miscarriages, however, occasionally indicate that there is some underlying genetic or autoimmune problem that warrants an in-depth medical workup.

Loss of the fetus after the first trimester affects about 5 percent of pregnancies. These losses are rarely caused by exposure to extremely high doses of a toxin (such as cocaine) or by a severe maternal infection that passes through the placenta to the fetus. The most common cause for a late-pregnancy loss (after the first trimester) is an incompetent cervix (a cervix that cannot stay closed and hold the fetus inside the uterus). An incompetent cervix has usually been injured in some way, either by surgery or by repeatedly opening it artificially, as with multiple abortions. In addition, women whose mothers took DES (diethylstilbestrol), an infertility drug used during the 1950s and 1960s, often have cervical changes that have been associated with the inability to carry a pregnancy to full term.

Unfortunately, the diagnosis of an incompetent cervix can be made only after a pregnancy has been lost in the second trimester. An incompetent cervix may be corrected in subsequent pregnancies by a surgical procedure called a cervical cerclage. Basically, this procedure involves placing a purse-string stitch (one that draws the cervical opening closed) around the cervix. The stitch is left in place until the fetus matures and then removed before the onset of labor. If you have an incompetent cervix and the stitch has been placed, it is best to avoid strenuous activity.

Induced Abortions

As the law currently stands, women in the United States still have the right to choose to terminate an unwanted pregnancy. This decision is an emotionally difficult one and should not be made without some type of counseling. Ideally, your regular health-care provider should be able to counsel you on this issue, but as you have a choice, so do practitioners: Some feel they don't have to perform abortions or refer or counsel anyone about their choices. If you cannot get any information from your own practitioner, you would be best served by calling the nearest women's health center or family planning clinic. Even if the health center does not perform abortions on its premises, its staff should be able to give you some names and numbers to call.

When you call a clinic that offers abortion services, the counselor may give you information concerning the procedure itself, its cost, and your state's particular legal requirements. In light of recent violence against clinics, many clinics will not give any information over the phone. Some require that you come to the clinic and have a pregnancy test before a referral will be made. Some states now require that minors obtain written consent for the procedure from one or both parents. Some states require a 24-hour waiting period from the time you are examined at the abortion center and sign the consent form to the time the abortion is performed. For those women who must travel long distances to obtain an abortion, this waiting period may add an additional burden. Therefore, some abortion centers help women obtain overnight lodging in the community.

When you arrive at the health center, you will meet with a counselor who will discuss your decision with you, describe the procedure, and perform (or introduce you to the health-care provider who will) a physical examination. It is very important to know exactly how far along you are in your pregnancy. Abortions that are performed between 7 and 10 weeks from the first day of your last period involve the fewest serious medical complications (approximately 1 to 2 per 1,000 procedures). At any time between 10 to 12 weeks, there is a slightly higher risk of complication (3 per 1,000 procedures). At 13 to 14 weeks, the procedure becomes technically more difficult to perform and is associated with a greater chance of complications (6 per 1,000 procedures).

First-trimester abortions (up to 12 weeks after conception) can easily be performed in an outpatient setting. They may be performed under general anesthesia or with local anesthesia (like *Novocain*) injected into the cervix. Sometimes the local anesthesia is enhanced by intravenous sedation and/or pain relievers. The cervix is then gently dilated, and the pregnancy is removed with a suction curette. You can expect some bleeding and cramping after the procedure; the bleeding usually stops after two or three days, and the cramping can be relieved with ibuprofen. Two of the most common complications include fever and bleeding, both of which can be readily treated. If you experience a fever over 100.4°F, or if your bleeding is much heavier than a heavy period, you should call the clinic or your health-care provider. They can prescribe antibiotics for infection and drugs that stimulate uterine contraction. The drugs contract the uterine muscle, causing constriction of the blood vessels, and the bleeding then usually stops.

Abortions performed for pregnancies after the thirteenth week are more complex and usually require either hospital care or clinics that offer specialized services. The complication rate runs between 13 and 25 of every 1,000 pregnancies. Some states place restrictions on abortions performed during the second trimester, sometimes only allowing them for genetic problems or if the health and life of the mother are in danger.

RU 486

RU 486 is a drug that can induce abortion when taken soon after the first missed period and up to seven weeks after conception. A second medication is usually given in conjunction with RU 486, and both should be administered under the auspices of a trained health-care provider. When used properly, RU 486 can effectively induce abortions in 96 percent of cases. This drug has been safely and widely used in France and China, and drug trials of RU 486 may soon begin in the United States.

Unwanted pregnancies are always difficult, whether you are 15 or 45 years old. Involving your partner (and/or parent) in the difficult decision-making process is desirable but not always possible. Seeking emotional help from a friend, counselor, social worker, or therapist can be very helpful. Try not to go it alone. Carrying a pregnancy to term and giving the baby up for adoption, raising an unwanted child, or terminating a pregnancy are all terribly painful choices, and each carries its own long-term emotional burdens. Whatever decision you make, consider the choices carefully. After the decision is made, reevaluate your birth control options. Current contraceptive choices are far from perfect, but try to choose a contraceptive that is least likely to place you in the position of facing an unwanted pregnancy.

9

COMMON INFECTIONS

Some infections that affect women are not necessarily associated with sexual activity. Although they may flare up after sexual activity, they are not considered to be sexually transmitted diseases.

YEAST INFECTIONS

One of the most common infections affecting the vaginal and cervical tissue is a yeast infection caused by the fungus *Candida albicans*. Most women at some point in their lives experience a yeast infection. Although the symptoms are very uncomfortable, it is an infection that is easily treated in most women.

The normal, healthy vagina is acidic by nature. It is this acidity that prevents bacteria and fungi from developing into serious infections and inflammations. When something changes the pH (acid/base balance) of the vagina, making it more of an alkali (base) environment, the yeast spores that are ever present in the vagina grow rapidly and cause the irritating symptoms. The action is similar to that of bread yeast, which will grow rapidly once you add sugar to the bread dough.

Several things can change the pH balance of the vagina from acidic to alkali. Eating lots of sugar or yeasty foods (including beer) is one example. This is why many women get yeast infections around the holidays, when they eat more baked goods. Taking antibiotics will often change the pH of the vagina by destroying the normal balance of bacteria, thereby enabling the normal numbers of vaginal yeast to proliferate and create an infection. Diabetics, who have higher blood sugar, are more prone to yeast infections. Pregnant women also have an increased incidence of yeast infections. The birth control pill itself puts women into a state of pseudopregnancy, and some women have a slightly increased risk of developing yeast infections while on the Pill, although this is less common with the low-dose pills used today.

Another factor that will make the vagina more susceptible to yeast infections is increased moisture and heat that normally surround the vagina. Women should avoid wearing a wet bathing suit or exercise leotard for an extended amount of time, especially if it is made out of spandex or heavy Lycra, which does not allow air to reach the vagina. Fungus thrives in moist, dark, warm places.

Symptoms

The symptoms of yeast infections vary widely but usually start with mild discomfort and itching of the labia, noticed at first when a woman wipes herself after urinating. Shortly after that, she notices a burning sensation during urination, along with a white discharge is present. This discharge has copious curds (looking a little like cottage cheese), or it may have little or none at all. If left untreated, the itching often increases and the labia begin to swell and get quite red and painful to the touch. This may become very uncomfortable, to the point where it hurts to walk or sit down.

Treatment

In most instances, yeast infections are very easy to diagnose. In many cases, if you call your health-care provider and describe the symptoms, he or she will be able to advise you over the phone and suggest an over-the-counter remedy such as miconazole (*Monistat*) or clotrimazole (*Gyne-Lotrimin*). This is beneficial to you in a few ways. First, it will save you the cost of an office visit, which can range from $30 to $75 in a private practice. Then it will allow you to start the treatment without waiting for an appointment. The sooner the treatment gets started, the sooner the relief. Having to wait a day or more to be seen by the practitioner can mean a few extra days of symptoms. The worse a yeast infection gets, the longer it takes to get relief.

Some practitioners will insist on seeing you before making a diagnosis for the first time. They may prefer to see the clinical symptoms for themselves before prescribing a medication to treat the yeast. This may be especially true if the practitioner doesn't know you well or if the symptoms you describe are vague. A clinical diagnosis is made by evaluating the genitals with a speculum exam (which is never pleasant when you have a yeast infection) and by taking a small amount of the discharge and inspecting it under the microscope. Yeast spores and buds should be present and visible under the microscope. If there is any question about this, your practitioner should take a culture of the cervix and vagina to properly diagnose exactly what is causing your symptoms.

There are several commercial preparations for treatment of yeast infections. Some work better for some women than others, and they are usually prescribed according to your practitioner's preference.

Vaginal preparations.   The most common prescribed medications are creams or vaginal suppositories that are antifungals. The cream comes in a tube (like toothpaste) and has an applicator that screws on to the tube. When the tube is squeezed, the applicator is filled and then unscrewed from the tube. The applicator is then placed inside your vagina, as far up as it will comfortably go, and the plunger of the applicator is pushed to deposit the cream in the vagina. This is very similar to the insertion of a tampon. Instructions with diagrams accompany the cream. The cream is used at bedtime for one, three, or seven consecutive nights, depending on the preparation. Using the cream at bedtime will ensure that it stays inside the vagina for several hours. During the day the cream will slowly ooze out, and you may have to make several trips to the bathroom to wipe away the excess. Wearing a minipad is not really recommended, as the fiber or deodorizing chemicals in it tend to irritate the labia even more. Be sure to wear only cotton underwear—synthetic fibers do not allow air to circulate and thus make the problem worse.

The cost of the cream can be rather expensive, depending on where you buy it. The treatment can cost anywhere from $20 to $30, and if an office visit is added to this, a common yeast infection could cost you as much as $90 to treat. This is bad news for women who get such infections frequently. There are several home remedies for yeast infections; some, of course, work much better than others but, again, every woman responds differently. These treatments, as well as the commercial treatments, are safe to use during pregnancy.

Oral medications.   There are several oral medications that can be used for recurrent or resistant yeast infections. Nystatin pills (450,500 units daily for three to four weeks) may reduce systemic yeast, though they are less effective for vaginal yeast. Ketokonizol has been used for yeast, but it has been associated with some changes in liver enzymes and is infrequently used for vaginal yeast. Fluconizole (or *Diflucan*) (150 mg taken in a single dose) is the newest treatment for resistant/recurrent yeast. It seems to be a very effective treatment for vaginal yeast, unfortunately this single dose costs approximately $20.

Mild vinegar douches.   This very inexpensive treatment works quite well to relieve the symptoms of a yeast infection but often fails to cure it completely. If you have a douche bag, household vinegar, and cool water, it certainly is worth a try. You simply add one tablespoon of vinegar to a douche bag, fill it with cool tap water, and irrigate the vagina. This helps to wash away the yeast that is there and creates more of an acid environment. This should be done twice a day. The first few times may burn a bit—vinegar is an acid, and acid burns when the tissue is irritated. Still, one tablespoon of vinegar will not do any damage to the tissue. Most of the commercial preparations burn, too.

Yogurt. Homemade yogurt contains a bacillus that will kill yeast spores, and this may be used as a vaginal treatment. (Commercial yogurt, on the other hand, tends to contain added milk solids that could actually encourage yeast growth.) Homemade yogurt is also inexpensive and works well for some women. It is a little more difficult to get the yogurt into the vagina, but it can be done. The application is most easily accomplished by using your finger, scooping up a little (plain, unsweetened) yogurt, and inserting it into the vagina. Doing this three or four times should povide enough yogurt to be therapeutic. The applications should also be done at bedtime so that they stay in the vagina longer. Yogurt is very soothing for the symptoms and does not burn. Some people believe it is also beneficial for a woman to increase the amount of yogurt in her diet during a yeast infection, because yogurt reduces the amount of yeast spores in the gastrointestinal tract. If you are unfortunate enough to be plagued with recurring yeast infections, you should consider eating at least one serving of yogurt a day.

Boric acid. Boric acid suppositories are a safe and very effective way to treat yeast infections. They are also very inexpensive, and no prescription is needed. Boric acid is sold as a powder and can be found in a drugstore. You will also need to purchase size 0 gelatin capsules, which can be obtained from the pharmacist or at a health food store. These are usually sold in boxes of 100 and cost a couple of dollars. You simply fill the capsules with the boric acid powder and use them as suppositories. One capsule inserted into the vagina before bed for three consecutive nights should cure the yeast infection. You can use this method for as many nights as needed, since boric acid is very mild (it is used as an eyewash). The capsule will melt during the night, and the next day you will have a small amount of watery, gritty discharge. Most women do not find this discharge as bothersome as the creamy discharge. It should be noted that boric acid is toxic if taken orally. Never take the capsules by mouth, and be sure to keep boric acid out of the reach of children.

Most women get a yeast infection once or twice a year, more commonly around the holidays, or in the humid days of summer. There are some women, though, who get them repeatedly, and this can be very disruptive to their lives. Those who suffer from chronic yeast infections should see a health-care provider for a complete physical. A screening test for diabetes should be done, too, because chronic yeast is one of the warning signs of diabetes. Yeast infections are also common in people who are immunosuppressed, such as AIDS and leukemia patients, so a complete physical is really critical if the infection occurs four to six times a year.

It is very uncommon for two heterosexual partners to pass yeast back and forth, but it is not impossible. If a male partner is not circumcised, he may be harboring the yeast spores under the foreskin and reinfecting his partner during intercourse. This is not at all common in circumcised males, since yeast tends to wash off very easily in the shower. A woman who harbors an excessive amount of yeast in her vagina may find that the friction of intercourse is just enough to bring on a full-blown yeast infection. This does not mean she is getting the yeast from her partner. One remedy that may be very helpful in a case like this is for the woman to use one dose of a yeast treatment following each act of intercourse. It also may help to use either a commercial cream for treating yeast or a bit of plain yogurt as a lubricant before intercourse. Saliva, which is acidic, makes a very good lubricant, and lubrication is the key here. Without proper lubrication, the friction of intercourse is much more irritating, and a yeast infection is much more likely to ensue. The transmission of yeast is more common among lesbians because the vagina is a more hospitable environment for yeast.

Prevention

There are a number of ways a woman can prevent yeast infections:

1. Eat a healthy diet, and avoid too many sweets or yeasty foods such as breads, beer, and wine. Include yogurt as a source of calcium and protein.
2. Wear only cotton underwear, or no underwear at all.

3. Make sure you have adequate lubrication before sexual intercourse.
4. Take antibiotics only when necessary.
5. Change out of a wet bathing suit or sweaty exercise wear as
   soon as possible.

URINARY TRACT INFECTIONS

A urinary tract infection (UTI) is a very uncomfortable and painful
condition. If left untreated, it can become truly serious, and in rare
circumstances it may be life-threatening. Fortunately, this is an infection that is easily treated with antibiotics. The vast majority of women
will not let a UTI go untreated, because the symptoms become so
severe that activities of daily living become impossible. Rarely, however, a woman will have a UTI without noticing any pain at all. This
happens more commonly during pregnancy, so it is important to be
aware of the accompanying symptoms and to treat the infection
quickly.

Human liquid waste (urine), unlike solid waste (feces), should contain no bacteria. Under normal circumstances, it is a sterile substance.
This is not true of feces, which are loaded with bacteria. When bacteria get into the urethra and up into the bladder, a urinary tract infection results. The most common bacterial cause of a UTI is *Escherichia
coli (E. coli)*, which usually enters the bladder from the skin around the
anus. This can happen in a number of ways. The urethra, which is the
passageway for the elimination of urine, is just above the vagina and
not far from the anus. When wiping the area after urinating or defecating, it is easy for bacteria from the anal area to be introduced into
the urethra. The bacteria then travel up the short urethra and into the
bladder. It is for this reason that girls should be taught as soon as they
are toilet trained to wipe from front to back. This simple instruction
will greatly reduce the chances of getting a UTI during childhood and
much later on as well. Boys and men, because of their anatomy, are far
less likely to be afflicted with a UTI. The opening to their urethra at

the end of the penis is much farther away from the rectum. The male's urethra is also longer than the female's, and the bacteria have farther to travel before reaching the bladder. En route to the bladder, bacteria are flushed out by simply urinating. Therefore, the greater distance to the bladder does make a difference. Males also have the advantage of not having to wipe themselves each time after urinating.

Symptoms

The symptoms of a UTI usually start with little more than a frequent urge to urinate. When you do urinate, though, only a small amount of urine comes out. This is generally followed by a sensation of pressure bearing down as you empty your bladder. Abdominal cramps and backache are often next, followed by a strong burning sensation during urination. You may also notice that the urine is pinkish, which means there is some blood in it. There may be a strong odor, too. The symptoms can rapidly progress and become generalized to the point where you feel like you've got the flu. You are achy and feverish, and the thought of using the toilet again makes you nauseated.

A history of the above symptoms requires immediate medical attention. A call to your practitioner is warranted because you need to have a laboratory test done and an antibiotic prescribed. The trip to the lab will entail a urinalysis and a urine culture and antibiotic sensitivity tests. You will be provided with towelettes and asked to clean your urethral area, to urinate a little bit into the toilet, and then to urinate into a sterile container. This is called midstream, "clean catch" urine. It is collected in this fashion to avoid getting labial bacteria into the urine and making the results less accurate. The practitioner wants to see if bacteria are present in the urine. It involves a lab technician preparing the urine sample and examining it under the microscope. The presence of bacteria or blood in the urine would indicate a UTI. The urinalysis can be accomplished in a half hour or less, and your practitioner can decide to treat you based on the results.

The urine culture and antibiotic sensitivity tests take longer. The urine is placed in a specific culture medium and kept at 37°C for 24 to 48 hours. The bacteria will grow on the culture medium, and the specific organism can then be identified. The laboratory will also be able to tell exactly which antibiotic the bacteria are sensitive to. This test gives much more accurate information than just a urinalysis and, therefore, the treatment can be more specific. The problem with this test is that it takes a full 48 hours for the bacteria to grow. A woman with severe symptoms should never wait that long for treatment. By that time, the infection could have traveled upward from the bladder to the kidneys, creating a much more critical situation. Most physicians will treat immediately, then change the antibiotic if necessary when the culture results are known.

Diabetics have a higher incidence of urinary tract infections because they have sugar in their urine, an environment in which bacteria thrive. Diabetics in good control (who don't have urinary glucose) still run a high risk for UTIs.

Pregnant women also have a higher risk of getting a UTI. As the fetus grows in the uterus, it deprives the bladder of space to expand and may inhibit a total emptying of the bladder during urination. When urine stagnates in the bladder, there is more opportunity for bacteria to flourish.

Sexual intercourse itself does not cause UTIs, but it is frequently a co-factor. The friction of the penis against the top wall of the vagina (where the urethra is) can increase the chance of vulvar organisms passing into the bladder. If there is contamination from the rectum, as with anal intercourse followed by vaginal intercourse, it is far more likely that a UTI will ensue. In postmenopausal women, the outer third of the urethra can thin and cause frequent UTIs, especially after intercourse. These problems are diminished in women taking estrogen-replacement therapy.

An ill-fitting diaphragm, especially one that is too large, can also cause urinary tract infections. When the rim of the diaphragm restricts the urethra, the urine is retained in the bladder and the risk of a UTI increases.

Women who have abnormally short or narrow urethras are also at a higher risk for a UTI. With a short urethra, bacteria do not have far to go before reaching the bladder and will not often be flushed out in time. With a narrow urethra or one obstructed with polyps, emptying of the bladder may not be adequate.

Treatment

The treatment for all urinary tract infections is an appropriate antibiotic. There are broad-spectrum antibiotics that will kill a wide range of bacteria, but with the overuse of antibiotics, many bacteria have become resistant. The penicillins are effective against some organisms, but these will cause a yeast infection in many women. Your health-care provider must ascertain whether you have an allergy to any specific antibiotic. Therefore, it is crucial that you let your practitioner know if you've had a reaction to any medication you've ever taken. If you have had a reaction to penicillin, you should never be given any antibiotic from that group. With all the new antibiotics being produced, your practitioner should be able to find one to which you are not sensitive.

The sulfa drugs, especially in combination with trimethoprim (*Bactrim, Septra*), are effective against UTIs and are stronger, so they don't need to be taken as frequently as the penicillins. Nitrofurantoin (*Macrodantin*) is an antibiotic specifically for the bladder that works very effectively against UTIs. This drug will not cause a yeast infection. Quinolones (*Norfloxacin, Ciprofloxacin,* and *Ofloxacin*) are also widely used. Cephalosporins (*Keflex, Velocef*) may also be effective in treating UTIs.

Phenazopyridine (*Pyridium*) is not an antibiotic but an antispasmodic that will numb the bladder and make it more comfortable during urination until the antibiotic resolves the symptoms. Your practitioner may prescribe this for you; if he or she does not, you may certainly ask for it. The drug is taken only for a day or two to get you through the worst of your symptoms. It will probably turn your urine a very dark orange, and it may be frightening the first few times you urinate and see what looks like bloody urine.

Apart from these and other medications, there are many things you can do for yourself when you first start to feel the symptoms of a UTI. First and foremost, drink lots of fluids. This is the most important thing you can do. Take in water as fast as you can. It will cause you to urinate more (which is an unpleasant thought), but you will be flushing the bacteria out of your bladder. Making the urine more acidic will help kill the bacteria. Cranberry juice, vitamin C (ascorbic acid), and plain aspirin will help make the bladder more acidic, and therefore less hospitable for bacterial growth.

Rest and try to reduce your stress level if you can. If you are running around busily doing errands and attending meetings, you will not be able to drink the amount of fluids needed or to empty your bladder as often.

Empty your bladder as soon as you feel the urge. Holding urine for an extended amount of time will predispose you to a UTI if you don't already have one. Don't stray too far from a bathroom.

Empty your bladder as soon as possible after intercourse to flush out the bacteria that may be creeping up the urinary tract. If you drink a glass of water before having sex, you should be able to urinate afterward. And never follow anal penetration with vaginal penetration unless your partner gets up to wash in between. Anal penetration without washing will make you more susceptible to urinary tract infections and to vaginal infections as well.

If you have recurrent UTIs, reduce the amount of alcohol you consume. Heavy alcohol intake will exacerbate your risk of recurrent infection.

Try taking vitamin C (500 milligrams) every morning and night. It may help to reduce the risk of recurrent UTIs.

Always, always wipe from front to back to avoid introducing bacteria from the rectum into the urethra.

If you are pregnant, waste no time in seeking treatment for urinary symptoms. Even if you are only urinating frequently and have a backache, call your practitioner immediately. An untreated UTI in pregnancy can lead to premature labor and a miscarriage. UTIs are not something to be taken lightly in pregnancy.

BACTERIAL VAGINOSIS

Bacterial vaginosis is the most recent name applied to the extremely common bacterial vaginal infection previously known as nonspecific vaginitis, *Hemophilus vaginalis,* or *Gardnerella.* Various bacteria can cause this infection, but the most common is *Gardnerella,* a bacterium that normally inhabits the gut. With the proximity of the anus and the vagina, it can sometimes invade the vagina, disturbing the normal balance of vaginal bacteria and thereby creating an infection. Other common bacteria causing bacterial vaginosis include *Streptococcus, Mobiluncus,* bacteroids, and *E. coli.*

Vaginal contamination may occur because of poor wiping procedure after urinating or defecating, or the bacteria may be transferred by sexual intercourse. Males who carry the organism may or may not have any symptoms. Because the infection may be passed along sexually, both partners may need to be treated when it is discovered. There is really no sound research proving that treatment of both partners reduces the all-too-common recurrence of the infection in women, but it makes sense, especially in recurrent infections.

Symptoms

In women, bacterial vaginosis is often characterized by a fishy-smelling vaginal discharge that may be yellow or gray-white in color and thin, watery, or frothy to creamy in texture. Other less common symptoms include vaginal burning, itching, or irritation. Sometimes the symptoms may be so mild you may not be aware of the infection. You (or your sexual partner) may notice only a slight difference in your vaginal odor. The same bacteria that cause bacterial vaginosis can also infect males. The symptoms in men include mild penile discharge and mild burning with urination, but may not be severe enough to warrant any suspicion.

Treatment

One treatment with very effective results involves taking an oral antibiotic for one week. One of the most commonly prescribed antibiotics is metronidazole (*Flagyl*) in a dose of either 500 milligrams twice a day or 250 milligrams three times a day for a week. It has recently been shown to be effective in a single oral dose of 2 grams. It should be noted that you must not drink alcohol when taking this antibiotic; it will induce vomiting. (Drug-induced vomiting after alcohol consumption is called the *Antabuse*—disulfiram—effect.) If you vomit the antibiotic, it cannot be absorbed at all. Clindamycin (*Cleocin*) is another effective antibiotic for bacterial vaginosis. This is more expensive than metronidazole, but does not have the *Antabuse* effect and can safely be taken in pregnancy. Metronidazole is not recommended during pregnancy, particularly in the first trimester. Clindamycin is taken in a dose of 300 milligrams twice a day for a week. Metronidazole is now also available as a vaginal gel, and clindamycin is also sold as a vaginal cream. These two preparations are currently the treatments of choice. These antibiotics are available only by prescription, so a visit to your health-care provider is essential. There are several other antibiotics that may be tried, but the two described above are by far the most effective.

Triple sulfa cream is sometimes prescribed for this infection, too, but it is ineffective and usually not worth the time and expense. The cream may alleviate symptoms while you are using it, but the symptoms almost always recur once the cream is discontinued.

Prevention

If you have a tendency to get recurrent bouts of bacterial vaginosis, a few things can be tried. First, be scrupulous about hygiene, especially after using the toilet. If you are sexually active, check with your sexual partner. Be sure he or she has been treated simultaneously and has been compliant with the treatment. Once you have eliminated those factors, you can use a regimen of boric acid. Fill number 0 gelatin capsules with boric acid powder and use them as suppositories. Insert one of the capsules into the vagina at bedtime every night for one week. This will encourage the growth of the normal acid-loving vaginal bacteria, which keep a healthy pH balance. You may repeat this treatment monthly during the week preceding your period. Sometimes a six-month regimen is needed to break the cycle of recurring infection. This is a safe, easy, and inexpensive way to treat it.

With all of these nonsexually transmitted vaginal infections, lifestyle and diet play an important role. If you are plagued by recurrent infections of any kind and have ruled out medical factors such as underlying diseases, you need to take a look at your daily activities and habits. Fatigue, stress, pollution, and lack of proper nutrients can put you at a much higher risk for recurrent infections. Evaluate your diet. If you have a job or family situation that is causing undue stress, take the time to set priorities and determine what is important to you.

10

SEXUALLY TRANSMITTED DISEASES (STDs)

The incidence of sexually transmitted diseases has risen dramatically over the last 20 years. In the United States, more than 13 million people are affected by STDs annually—men and women of all educational and economic backgrounds, homosexuals as well as heterosexuals, and sexually active people of every race and age group. Nearly one-third of these cases occur in teenagers, and they are particularly common in people who engage in nonmonogamous sex. The actual number of cases of sexually transmitted diseases can only be estimated, because many infections produce no symptoms and many infections go untreated. Many of these diseases are asymptomatic (present no symptoms), so they can be passed from one sexual partner to another. Despite a lack of immediate symptoms, some of them can produce long-lasting and devastating effects, particularly in women. Some of these infections can cause damage to the fallopian tubes, which can lead to infertility, tubal pregnancy, or years of chronic pelvic pain.

Other infections, especially venereal warts, are thought to cause changes in cervical cells that can predispose women to cervical cancer. Some STDs can be passed from a pregnant mother to her unborn child, causing major and sometimes untreatable or fatal problems for her baby.

ACQUIRED IMMUNE DEFICIENCY SYNDROME (AIDS)

AIDS is the most frightening and devastating of all of the sexually transmitted diseases. It is debilitating and always fatal. AIDS is caused by the human immunodeficiency virus (HIV), which destroys the body's ability to fight off infection. The AIDS patient thus becomes susceptible to opportunistic infections, i.e., those infections that could be fought off by a healthy person but that cause severe illness in a person whose immune system is compromised.

HIV has been found in many body fluids, including tears and saliva, but seems to be transmissible only through the transfer of blood, semen, breast milk, or vaginal fluids. This is why intravenous drug users who share needles and people who have more than one sexual partner (or whose partner has more than one partner) are particularly at risk for contracting HIV. It can take up to six months from the time a person is infected with the AIDS virus until the time a blood test will show a marker for the infection.

The average time between infection with the virus and the first obvious symptoms of AIDS is ten years. It is during this latency period that people may seem perfectly healthy, even though they are carrying the virus and potentially spreading it to their sexual partners.

The dreadful social stigma attached to this disease has allowed people with HIV/AIDS to suffer not just from the disease but also from discrimination by employers, landlords, insurance companies, and others. Because the two groups that initially showed the highest incidence of the disease—male homosexuals and intravenous drug users—were considered by many to be on the fringes of society, some people erroneously assumed that other groups were not at risk of contracting

AIDS. A full decade of mistaking AIDS for a "them" disease and not an "us" disease has allowed for its social stigmatization and has probably reduced the ability of AIDS education programs to be seriously implemented. If you think you are not at risk for AIDS, then you have automatically increased your chances for contracting the disease.

In 1990 there was a 29 percent increase in the number of new cases reported in heterosexual women, making them the fastest-growing AIDS population. This compares with an increase of 18 percent for males during the same period. This slower rise in new cases among men reflects the AIDS awareness programs and concomitant protection efforts among homosexual males. Women do not seem to be taking these lessons to heart and do not adhere to those measures that are required to prevent the spread of this deadly disease. The 1990 figures showed more than 4,000 AIDS cases among women (which equals a rate of 4.3 per 100,000). By 1993 more than 85,000 women were suspected of carrying HIV in the United States. By the year 2000, if this trend continues, the number of cases in women and in men will be equal.

Symptoms

The symptoms of AIDS in women may be more vague than those that have been recognized for men. In fact, women have been diagnosed much later in the course of the disease, and many of the diagnostic criteria originally established for gay men and intravenous drug users have not proved applicable for women. Delayed diagnosis in women has led to delayed treatment and a more rapid progression of the disease. Diagnostic standards for women are only now being formulated.

General symptoms of AIDS include unexplained weight loss, rash, anemia, atypical pneumonia, fatigue, fever, diarrhea, joint pains, numbness and/or tingling in the hands and legs, shingles (herpes zoster), multiple and/or recurrent vaginal infections, yeast infections of the mouth and/or vagina, venereal wart infections unresponsive to usual treatment, recurrent oral and genital herpes infections, and Pap smears that detect rapidly progressive cervical dysplasia. Obviously, having a yeast infection does not mean that you are at risk for being diagnosed with AIDS. But because many of the symptoms are vague and commonplace, multiple combinations of these symptoms should make you and your health-care provider consider the possibility that you may have AIDS.

Diagnosis of the AIDS virus is made by detecting the antibody to HIV in the bloodstream. Researchers initially reported that within six weeks of exposure, 60 percent of all infected people would have developed an antibody response. Within three months of exposure, this figure would rise to 90 percent, and within six months, almost 100 percent of people would test positive for AIDS antibodies. But newer information seems to indicate that most people will develop an antibody response within six weeks, and nearly 100 percent will have done so within three months of exposure. A simple blood test using the ELISA (enzyme-linked immunosorbent assay) method for screening viral antibodies is the initial screening method. Because this test can come up positive in the presence of some other confounding disease processes (such as cirrhosis of the liver, kidney dialysis, or intravenous drug use), a second, more specific test (the Western blot test) is performed on all positive ELISA samples. Only if both tests are positive will a person be told that he or she is HIV-positive.

The hallmarks of an adequate HIV-testing program are pretest counseling, confidentiality, and then post-test counseling. Pretest counseling should include information about the disease, its patterns of spread and the behaviors associated with it, risk-reduction behaviors, the course of the disease, and the present methods of treatment. There should also be a discussion about the meaning of the HIV test, and what a negative or positive result means. No one should ever just nonchalantly walk into a testing center for an AIDS test without first thoroughly considering what he or she would actually do if told of a positive result.

Before contemplating a pregnancy, all women of childbearing age should consider their relationships with previous and current sexual partners as well as those partners' sexual and intravenous drug practices. Between 20 percent and 35 percent of all fetuses contract the AIDS virus from their HIV-positive mothers (whether the mothers are asymptomatic carriers of HIV or have full-blown AIDS). Taking AZT in pregnancy significantly reduces the risk of passing the HIV virus to the fetus in pregnancy. *All* women must consider AIDS testing, especially if they think they may be at risk. If a woman is already pregnant, she should consider being tested early in her pregnancy so that she may adequately evaluate all her medical options. HIV positive women should not breast feed, since the virus can be passed through breast milk.

AIDS testing may not be performed without your consent, and you should have a thorough understanding of its implications. If the test is negative but recent exposure is a real possibility, then the test should be repeated after six weeks and once again after three months to rule out the negative testing window that can occur during the latency period. If all three tests are negative, counseling should stress behavioral changes that can reduce a woman's risk for contracting the disease. If either test is positive, then counseling must include a review of the meaning of the test, the treatments available during the symptom-free years prior to the development of AIDS, support systems available in the community, the importance of having one's partners tested, and safer-sex practices required to protect an HIV-negative partner.

Treatment

There is presently no cure for AIDS. The best and only effective tool for limiting the spread of this disease is prevention. HIV treatment is broken down into two phases. The first phase is treatment and care of the HIV-positive person who has not shown any signs of the disease; the second phase is the care of the person with AIDS who has multiple medical, social, and psychological problems and is susceptible to succumbing to any one of a number of opportunistic diseases. Although new drug regimens are being formulated for both phases of the disease, at this point azidothymidine (AZT) or related drugs such as didanosine (DDI) and zalcitabine (*Hivid* or ddC) or d4T and combinations of these and other drugs are the recommended treatments for a person who is HIV-positive. There is also a new class of drugs being investigated called protease inhibitors, which may become effective, especially in combination, in preventing AIDS. For women, more frequent Pap smears (every three to six months) are recommended, since HIV-positive women are more prone to rapidly progressive cervical changes leading to cervical cancer. Emotional support and long-term planning for persons with AIDS (PWAs), their family members, care partners, and significant others should be part of the health-care plan. Once a person has exhibited symptoms, medical treatment will be aimed at specific infections, diseases, and cancers associated with AIDS. At this stage, emotional support and financial and logistical planning become even more essential to the treatment program. AIDS has no cure; right now our only hope is AIDS prevention.

The key to prevention is practicing safer sex and eliminating situations in which blood, semen, vaginal secretions, or breast milk from an HIV-positive person could be transmitted to a person without HIV. Safer sex includes abstaining from casual sex and engaging in sex only with a monogamous partner. In addition, condoms or dental dams should be regularly used if there is more than one partner or if the partner is at risk for AIDS. Both partners should feel free to discuss any sexual relationships they have ever had, their exposure to blood in the workplace or elsewhere, any past or present intravenous drug use, and their most recent HIV test results. This will help each person evaluate the risk factors.

Obviously, intravenous drug use is not a healthful practice. Using unbleached needles or sharing blood-contaminated needles increases the risks of contracting and spreading the AIDS virus. The core of AIDS prevention is not just free clean needles or free bleach to kill the virus before the needle is reused (although those interventions do help) but also drug treatment programs that address the addiction and the despair that lead to intravenous drug use. It is the cessation of intravenous drug use and not merely the reduction of possible blood exposure during drug use that will eventually limit the spread of AIDS.

Similarly, it is the emphasis on responsible, monogamous sex that is the basis of safer-sex practices. The use of latex male condoms or polyethylene female condoms will reduce the transmission of HIV. When used for every sexual act, condoms can prevent pregnancy 90 percent of the time. This implies that 10 percent of the time, condoms fail to prevent not only the passage of sperm but also disease-causing organisms such as HIV. The proper use of condoms should be an essential part of any AIDS-prevention program and is indeed integral to the concept of safer sex. Condoms do help prevent the spread of AIDS and other sexually transmitted diseases, but they are no substitute for responsible sexual choices.

CHLAMYDIA

Chlamydia is the most prevalent sexually transmitted disease in the United States today. Although there are no mandatory reporting policies regarding chlamydial infections, it is estimated that at least 3 million to 4 million cases occur each year. That is between 2 and 10 times the rate of total gonorrhea cases. In addition, there has been a logarithmic rise in the incidence of chlamydia in the last 10 years.

The organism *Chlamydia trachomatis,* which causes this infection, is classified as a bacterium even though it shares many properties with viruses. Chlamydiae, like bacteria, have a cell wall, and they reproduce by dividing in half. The cell wall allows the use of antibiotics in its treatment, since all antibiotics work by attacking bacterial cell walls. Like viruses, however, chlamydiae can live only within the cells of a person's organs, which means that culturing is very difficult and very expensive. The tests that are widely available for chlamydia are affordable, but they are neither as sensitive nor as specific as necessary. In 5 to 15 percent of cases, the tests will confirm a chlamydial infection when none is actually present; in 10 to 25 percent of cases, the tests miss the diagnosis even when the person is infected.

Symptoms

An even more difficult problem is knowing which women to culture and treat, because between 50 to 70 percent of women harboring this organism are asymptomatic. If symptoms *do* occur, they usually appear within one to three weeks from the time of exposure. The symptoms may include a yellow or yellowish-white vaginal discharge; vaginal spotting, especially after intercourse; pain with urination; and/or mild lower abdominal or pelvic discomfort. The pain usually starts out as mild or dull and gradually increases in intensity. Sometimes there is mild discomfort during intercourse. A male partner may also have no symptoms, but if he has a discharge of pus from the penis, pain with urination, and pain or swelling of the testicles, both partners should suspect that a chlamydia infection may be present. Both should be tested and treated. Anal intercourse with an infected partner can lead to infection. That symptomatic infection is called proctitis (inflammation of the anal canal and rectum).

A newborn may contract chlamydia when passing through the infected birth canal of the mother. The organism can infect the eyes, causing conjunctivitis (which can lead to blindness), and may infect the lungs, causing chlamydial pneumonia. If a child older than a newborn has symptoms of genital or anal infection and tests positive for chlamydia, then sexual abuse must be strongly suspected.

Diagnosis of the infection is best determined by a person's overall risk for chlamydia. If you have had more than one male sexual partner or you suspect that your partner has had more than one sexual partner, you are at greater risk. If you have multiple partners and you do not consistently use condoms (or at least some form of barrier contraception), you are at increased risk. If you are at risk and your health-care provider finds that your cervix bleeds easily when touched with a cotton swab, notices a large number of infection-fighting cells upon microscopic examination of your cervical mucus, or confirms a positive test for chlamydia, then both you and your partner should be treated. If you or your partner have a positive test for gonorrhea, each of you should be treated for both gonorrhea and chlamydia, since 30 to 50 percent of people with positive tests for gonorrhea will also be infected with chlamydia.

The most insidious consequence of chlamydial infections in women is pelvic inflammatory disease (PID). Up to 1 million women in the United States develop this serious infection each year. Although this disease is characterized by infection of the pelvic organs by differ-

ent kinds of organisms, chlamydia is often the one organism that
precipitates the infection. The infection encompasses the cervix,
uterus, and fallopian tubes and may severely damage those organs. If
the fallopian tubes become scarred, infertility may result; or if an egg
and sperm enter the scarred tubes, their progress may be impeded and
the fertilized egg may not make it to the uterus before it starts to grow
and become implanted. This results in a tubal (ectopic) pregnancy,
which leads to the death of the fetus and is a life-threatening complication for the mother.

Treatment

Chlamydia may be treated with antibiotics, and those of choice are
tetracycline or its close cousin, doxycycline (*Doryx, Vibramycin*), and a
new antibiotic, azithromycin (*Zithromax*). Another new antibiotic,
ofloxacin (*Floxin*), is very effective in the treatment of both chlamydia
and gonorrhea. Since these drugs are contraindicated during pregnancy, erythromycin (*ERYC, E-Mycin*) is necessary for pregnant
women as well as for people who cannot tolerate the other drugs.

Antibiotics should be taken for 7 to 10 days for infections limited
to the cervix or urethra and for 10 to 14 days for infections that are
suspected to be more widespread. Azithromycin provides the advantage of effecting a cure with a single high-dose regimen (1 gram in a
single dose).

If widespread infection is suspected, then an antibiotic injection (of
either ceftriaxone or cefoxitin) should be given before the start of the
10-to-14-day course of oral antibiotics. This will cover possible concomitant infection with gonorrhea and other bacteria that are suspected to cause PID. Both partners should be treated, and condoms
should be used throughout the treatment period. Rescreening for
chlamydia four to six weeks after treatment is recommended, since a
positive test at that time usually indicates that one or both people in
the relationship did not complete the full course of antibiotics or that
reinfection has already occurred. Treatment should also include safer-
sex counseling as well as testing for other STDs, such as gonorrhea and

syphilis. In addition, high-risk sexual behavior should be assessed to determine if HIV testing should be offered.

GENITAL WARTS

Genital warts (condyloma) are infections caused by the human papillomavirus (HPV). The HPV is a large family of related viruses that cause warty growths ranging from the common wart to plantar warts (found on the soles of the feet) to warty growths on the vocal cords (laryngeal polyps). The subtypes of this virus that cause genital warts are usually spread by sexual contact. There are at least 3 million new cases reported each year, but since at least half the people who are infected with the virus show no signs of infection, the actual number of cases is unknown. A recent study of 18-year-old women entering college showed that 69 percent of the study group tested positive for HPV. In addition, about 65 to 70 percent of the partners of HPV-infected people will eventually develop the infection. It is dangerous for affected women because it can predispose them to precancerous changes of the cervix, vagina, and external genitals.

Before any discussion of venereal warts can begin, it must be noted that the behavior of the wart virus is only now being elucidated. In fact, AIDS research has shed light on, and has the increased research into the behavior of many other viruses, including HPV. However, the more virology research reveals, the more we realize how little we truly knew before. Many concepts regarding the behavior of HPV are controversial. Therefore, it's likely that much of the information given by diverse health-care providers and found in various written sources will be contradictory.

Human papillomaviruses constitute a family of more than 60 closely related viruses. At least a dozen members (i.e., viral subtypes) of this family have been isolated from warts that have the capacity to grow in the genital region. Certain subtypes, like the ones commonly found in plantar warts, cannot be transmitted to the genital region, and vice versa. HPV is thought to be spread at the time the moist, infected skin of the genital region of one partner comes into contact with the genitals of his or her partner. In addition, men can also transmit the virus in their semen.

At the time of contact, the virus, which is encased in its protein coat during the transmission phase, attaches itself to the recipient's genital cells, then sheds its protein coat and inserts its genetic material into the recipient's cells. Once inside a cell, the viral DNA can multiply and spread to adjoining cells. This process may all go on asymptomatically.

A visible wart is produced only when the infected cell is stimulated and the virus multiplies over and over again. The stimulus for this spurt of viral growth is as yet unknown, but it appears that many factors may turn on the viral switch. These include physical stress (when you are run down from a bad cold, another infection, a medical problem like diabetes, for example), psychological stress, immune-related stress (when you are taking immunosuppressant drugs such as cortisone, or if you have a disease that involves the immune system such as lupus or AIDS), or chemical exposure (such as the semen of a new sexual partner).

Although the people at greatest risk for becoming infected with the wart virus are sexually active men and women who do not use condoms and who have multiple sexual partners, this virus has occasionally been isolated in people who claim to have never been sexually active. The mode of transmission in these cases has not been adequately explained.

Warts have two common types of appearances: (1) common warty growths called exophytic warts, which are seen on the vulva, in the urethra, and in the lower part of the vagina, and (2) flat warts seen only with the help of a mild vinegar solution, which tends to make them appear white. Genital warts are most often seen on the cervix and in the upper part of the vagina. Either type of wart may be found on the male genitals (on the scrotum, on the shaft and head of the penis, in the urethra, and in the rectal canal).

Rectal condyloma are commonly found in both men and women and need not be the result of anal intercourse. The wart virus can spread to the rectum from other infected genital cells and can actually form a viral reservoir even after intensive treatment of the genital area has been performed. It is therefore believed that this virus can never truly be expunged from the genital area no matter what form of treatment is used, because the virus infects the cells of the entire anal and genital area and only occasionally appears in small areas at a time.

Symptoms

Genital warts generally produce no pain and only rarely cause itching. If sufficiently large, they can bleed when irritated (such as with pressure from the seam of an undergarment or with wiping after urination). If the warts are external and of the exophytic type, you may feel them when wiping, when showering, or during sexual activity. Flat warts usually go undetected in women unless they are picked up on a Pap smear.

Unfortunately, many genital warts (usually of the flat variety) are seen only with the help of magnifying equipment. For men and women, the external genitals can be examined with a good light source and a powerful magnifying lens after the genitals have been soaked with a mild vinegar solution. For women, the vagina and cervix must be carefully inspected as well. The magnifying device used to examine women both internally and externally is called a colposcope, and the examination is called colposcopy. The colposcope itself is really just a pair of binoculars set on a stand with an intense and directed light source built in. It magnifies the anatomy of the vulva, vagina, and cervix so that any abnormalities will stand out. To be sure that the warty lesion is truly a wart and not some other problem, a biopsy of the most abnormal looking area is taken and sent to a pathology lab.

Because the presence of HPV is associated with precancerous and even cancerous changes of the cervix, vagina, and vulva, the biopsy will reveal if these changes are present or not. Although only about 20 percent of warts are associated with cancers or precancerous changes, 80 to 90 percent of cervical, vaginal, and vulvar precancers and cancers contain the wart virus. Because the flat warts are generally not visible to the naked eye, sexually active women should have yearly Pap smears to screen for HPV and any precancerous and cancerous changes that can accompany them. Since Pap smears can miss abnormal cells about 15 percent of the time, repeating the screening yearly will not allow these generally slow-changing cells to progress beyond the early treatable stages. In addition, only about 20 percent of the precancerous cells progress to cancer. The other 80 percent remain either as early precancers or are repaired by the body's immune system and revert to normal-appearing cells. This does not mean that the wart virus disappears altogether. It may only mean that the virus reverts to a dormant state from which it can again be activated or where it may rest indefinitely.

One of the biggest controversies today concerning the containment of this virus centers on the examination and treatment of male sexual partners. Until recently, it was felt that if the genital wart virus was found in a woman, her partner should be examined. Virologists also suspected that if a treated woman had sex with her partner, she would just be reinfected, a situation referred to as the "Ping-Pong effect." It is now believed that because the virus can never be totally eradicated from either partner, reinfection in a treated man or woman is most likely the reactivation of the already-present virus, rather than a new reinfection by a partner.

Men who have visible warts *should* be examined and treated, even though only rarely are the warts associated with precancerous or cancerous lesions of the penis. However, if a male partner has no visible warts, then he need not have to undergo examination of the genitals, urethra, and anal canal. Because this issue is still being discussed, many women who are undergoing extensive treatment for recurrent lesions feel more comfortable knowing their partner has been thoroughly examined by a qualified practitioner.

If you have a new partner, condoms should be worn to reduce the spread of most STDs. However, condoms afford only limited protection from the spread of condyloma, since the virus can be present on surfaces not covered by the condom.

Treatment

All women with precancerous changes associated with HPV are candidates for treatment. In the treatment of genital warts, the visible lesion is removed by chemicals, heat, electric current, cryotherapy (freezing at very low temperatures), surgical excision, or laser. Once the majority of the virus-infected tissue has been treated or removed, the immune system begins to heal the affected area and suppress further viral activity. Because the virus is still present in the surrounding tissue, warts can recur.

External warts are generally treated with chemical agents (podophyllin, bichloroacetic acid, or trichloroacetic acid). These create a chemical burn and must be washed off within four hours of application. Anytime a chemical agent is used to treat warts, the skin surrounding the wart should be carefully covered with petroleum jelly so that only the warty area is burned. This will reduce the discomfort caused by the treatment.

Usually, several weekly treatments are required to eradicate the warts. Podophyllin can be applied on a weekly basis by your health-care practitioner in his or her office. Although this medication requires a diagnosis and prescription from your practitioner, it is now available in a milder form that can be used in a self-treatment program for external warts. Podophyllin should not be used by pregnant women because it is toxic to the fetus.

Bichloroacetic and trichloroacetic acids are applied in the office by your health-care practitioner. Because they are more caustic, they cause a more intense chemical burn. This means that they will generally suppress the virus with fewer weekly applications, but each application may be more uncomfortable than an application of podophyllin. These two closely related acid treatments are considered safe for use in pregnancy.

External and internal warts can be burned off with an electrical instrument, but old-fashioned instruments resembling small hot pokers are rarely used today. Newer, more precise electrocautery loops are now standard. The surgical procedure that utilizes this instrument is known as LEEP (loop electrocautery excision procedure), in which titanium wires allow for precise excision of warty lesions. The loop can also be used to treat wart-related precancerous changes of the cervix diagnosed by Pap smear and colposcopy.

Cryotherapy (freezing) has been used for many years to treat both external and internal warts and the precancerous lesions with which they are associated. Cryotherapy burns the infected tissue when directed to the specific area for a long enough period, in much the way that dry ice will burn your fingers if held for any length of time. The burned area will slough off, and the immune system will stimulate the regeneration of new, healthy tissue. As with electrocautery, new warts may grow after cryotherapy, since the virus cannot be completely eradicated.

Surgical excision (cutting out wart-infected areas) does the same basic job as burning or freezing. It removes the most affected areas and stimulates the immune system to heal the area and suppress further viral activity. For small warty areas that have not responded to chemical treatment, surgical excision offers both the ability to remove the warts and the ability to obtain infected tissue to send to a pathology laboratory for accurate identification. This can be crucial when the affected area looks like a wart but in the end is only a wartlike growth not related to HPV. Surgical excision is rarely used anymore because loop excision and laser methods can remove affected tissue more precisely.

Laser is a form of light, and light is a form of electromagnetic energy. Surgical laser harnesses this energy so that it can be precisely directed to cut out a piece of virus-infected tissue deep within the body or to simply vaporize it if the area is superficial. The two most common types of laser used to treat warts are the carbon dioxide laser and the Yag laser. It must be remembered that laser is not magic; its basic function (like cautery, freezing, and surgical excision) is to remove the most obviously wart-infected or precancerous areas and to stimulate the immune system to heal the area and suppress further viral growth.

When done properly, all treatment choices have approximately the same cure rates. Wart suppression occurs in 80 to 90 percent of cases, usually for at least several months. With loop, cryotherapy, and laser, approximately 90 percent of precancerous changes caused by HPV can be cured. Since all of these methods involve burning, cutting, or vaporizing the skin, treatment of external warts can be very uncomfortable and, if extensive, extremely painful. Burning the external genital region will cause soreness and require good posttreatment care. Soaking in warm bath water is therapeutic, but balanced saltwater similar to ocean water is even better. This can be created in the bathtub with a special aquarium product, Instant Ocean, that is widely available. Topical burn creams combined with numbing creams are also used successfully after treatment. Internal treatments are not usually painful, but they can cause an uncomfortable vaginal discharge.

If you require treatment for the wart virus, ask your health-care provider what you may expect from the procedure regarding both its success rate in your particular case and the projected recuperation time. Be aware that the presence of the virus does not always require treatment, that the virus frequently recurs, and that it can seem to burn itself out and become inactive over several years. Understand that genital warts probably never disappear completely and that they have the potential of reappearing many months or years later.

GONORRHEA

Gonorrhea (also known as GC or the clap) is caused by a bacterium called *Neisseria gonorrheae*. Ninety percent of reported cases in women occur in women under age 30, and 25 percent are in women under age 20. Although the number of cases reported annually has stabilized at about 1 million per year, it is believed that probably at least another 1 million cases (mostly in teenagers) go unreported. In addition, a new problem has developed since 1976; the year the first cases of penicillin-resistant gonorrhea were identified. Since the development of penicillin in the early 1940s, gonorrhea was treated easily and inexpensively. However, with the onset of the newly resistant strains, new and more expensive drugs have had to be developed. Also, the threat of the prospect of newer drug-resistant strains of the bacterium looms ahead.

In women, gonorrhea infection usually initially occurs in the cervix, although it may cause infection in the throat, urethra, and/or rectum. The disease is spread by direct contact—from the genitals to the mouth, from the genitals to the anus, and from the genitals to the genitals. Moreover, it can be spread with moist fingers from the genitals to the mouth or anus. Contrary to many widespread stories, gonorrhea is not spread from contact with inanimate objects such as toilet seats.

Symptoms

Gonorrhea may be totally asymptomatic in 40 to 60 percent of women. Otherwise, symptoms include increased vaginal discharge, sore throat or tonsillitis, urinary burning or frequency, or rectal burning or itching. If symptoms do develop, they will usually be noticed between 2 to 10 days after sexual contact with an infected partner. If the initial site of infection is the cervix (whether symptomatic or not), gonorrhea can spread directly up to the uterus, fallopian tubes, and ovaries (causing pelvic inflammatory disease) or through the bloodstream to other parts of the body (causing infective arthritis and skin rash). Late-stage symptoms include pelvic and lower abdominal pain, joint pain, fever, and/or vomiting.

In men, the symptoms of gonorrhea usually include penile discharge (with or without urinary burning), rectal burning, and/or sore throat or tonsillitis. Newborn babies may contract gonorrhea after passing through the mother's infected birth canal. This can result in neonatal gonococcal eye infection, which if left untreated can lead to blindness. In most states, all newborns must receive treatment for this potential infection soon after birth. If an older child is found to have gonorrhea, there should be a very high suspicion of child sexual abuse, and a proper investigation should be done.

Diagnosis of gonorrhea can be made by culturing those areas that are most likely to be infected. If you suspect you may be at risk for gonorrhea, you must tell your health-care provider what sites may have been exposed to infection so that the proper cultures may be taken. If you allow shyness or embarrassment to interfere with your ability to communicate frankly with your care provider, you may be putting yourself at major risk.

For women, the long-term risks of gonorrhea, like those of chlamydia, include PID—the spread of infection to the uterus, fallopian tubes, and ovaries. Nevertheless, although gonorrhea and/or chlamydia can initiate this upward-spreading infection, many other bacteria contribute to the infection's damaging effects on the tubes and ovaries. This damage can lead to destruction of the tubes and to infertility in at least 10 percent of cases. Also, scarring of the tubes can cause impairment of tubal function. This in turn can impede the proper passage of a fertilized egg down the fallopian tube on its way to the uterus. If the fertilized egg then implants in the tube, the result is a tubal (ectopic) pregnancy that does not develop into a baby. Even the limited growth of an embryo in the tube can lead to tubal rupture and hemorrhage. Therefore, the damaged tube not only thwarts the growth of a potential pregnancy but can also endanger the life of the mother. And damaged pelvic organs can lead to a lifetime of intermittent or continuous pelvic pain.

Treatment

Penicillin is no longer recommended for the treatment of gonorrhea because of the exponential rise in the incidence of penicillin-resistant strains. Several antibiotics can be used to treat gonorrhea. Ceftriaxone (*Rocephin*) or spectinomycin (*Trobicin*) are given by injection. Ofloxacin (*Floxin*), ampicillin (*Omnipen*)/amoxicillin (*Amoxil*) plus probenecid (*Benemid*), or erythromycin (*ERYC, E-Mycin*) is given by mouth. Both sexual partners must be treated (even if one partner's culture is negative). A week after the completion of the antibiotic treatment, the partners should be recultured. If a person still tests positive after treatment, both partners should undergo another full treatment course and again be recultured. Because 30 to 50 percent of those people infected with gonorrhea are also infected with chlamydia, anyone who tests positive for either disease should be treated for both (as should their partner). Obviously, the best treatment is prevention. As with other sexually transmitted diseases, the way to avoid gonorrhea is through abstinence or a monogamous relationship. Otherwise, the regular use of condoms and spermicide is indispensable.

HERPES

Genital herpes infections are caused by the herpes simplex virus (HSV). This virus is extraordinarily common, affecting at least 30 million Americans. The number of new cases that occur annually is estimated to be at least half a million. Such a figure can only be estimated, because many people who are infected never exhibit any symptoms. Twenty percent of genital herpes cases are caused by the common oral herpes virus, Type I (HSV I). The other 80 percent are caused by Type II (HSV II). Oral herpes, which goes by the name of cold sores, fever blisters, or canker sores, is present in almost all adults, whether they have ever had any symptoms or not. It does not matter if it is Type I or Type II. If herpes is on the genitals, it is called genital herpes. Because oral-genital transmission of the two different subtypes occurs easily during oral sex, it is easy to see how this virus has become so widespread.

Herpes infections often appear as a group of tiny, whitish blisters or ulcerations, each surrounded by a reddish rim. They can be painful or itchy. Sometimes, however, they just look like a small but painful patch of broken skin on the external genitals. The appearance of herpes can vary so widely that identifying and diagnosing it can prove to be very difficult. This in turn contributes to underestimating the number of genital herpes cases in the United States.

Herpes can be found on the external genitals or in the urethra (in both men and women), in the vagina, on the cervix, in the folds of the groin skin, on the buttocks, or at the base of the spine. If it is present on the cervix or in the vagina, it may not produce any symptoms or any visible lesions. Although it seems more likely that the infection is spread at the time of an outbreak of open sores, herpes can also be spread by a sexual partner who is a carrier of the virus but who has had no visible signs at all. Like most viruses, herpes lives within the cells of the person who carries the virus, and it can only be passed from the mucous membranes of one person to those of another. It cannot be passed by casual contact or from contact with inanimate objects such as toilet seats.

Symptoms

The first infection with herpes may produce no symptoms at all; or it can involve classic symptoms of a serious primary infection. These classic symptoms usually occur between 2 to 10 days from the time of initial viral exposure. The first sign is local burning or itching, soon followed by a widespread outbreak of red bumps that progress to painful blisters and then to open sores or ulcers. The sores crust over and slowly resolve during the next 10 days to 2 weeks. The total length of the initial outbreak is generally 2 to 3 weeks, but it may last as long as 3 to 6 weeks. If the sores are in or around the urethra, a woman may find it so painful to urinate that she becomes unable to empty her bladder. In severe cases, this leads to involuntary urinary retention and requires catheterization of the bladder and sometimes even hospitalization until the pain of urination diminishes.

The classic primary infection is often accompanied by fever, loss of appetite, joint pains and muscle aches, headache, swollen glands all over the body (especially in the groin), and a feeling of general malaise. If these are the only symptoms present and are not accompanied by the outbreak of genital blisters, they could easily be mistaken for any flu-like viral infection.

Once the virus has established itself, with or without symptoms, it withdraws from the genital areas and travels up the sensory nerves to the nerve cells in the spinal cord, where it quietly resides in an inactive state. When roused from its dormant state, it will travel back down the sensory nerves to the genitals. There, it multiplies and can be contagious, even when no genital blisters, sores, or fissures have erupted. If blisters and sores do appear, they tend to be less widespread than they were before, lasting for only a total of a week to 10 days. The frequency and timing of these recurrent outbreaks vary widely from person to person. Some people get only a few symptomatic outbreaks over many years, whereas others are plagued by frequent bouts of recurrent blisters. What triggers the virus from its quiescent state to its active state is unknown, but stress is thought to play a big part. Stress may be related to emotions, physical health (when you are tired and run down or have a serious illness like pneumonia, the flu, or uncontrolled diabetes), or the immune system (especially if it is suppressed by medications such as cortisone or by diseases such as lupus or AIDS).

Some people have felt devastated by a diagnosis of genital herpes. Women report feeling dirty, ashamed, or even suicidal. This response is absolutely out of proportion to the nature of what is really only a cold sore. Besides being intermittently painful or uncomfortable, this virus is more of a nuisance than a real medical problem.

The real medical danger posed by this infection occurs during pregnancy. The herpes virus may infect a child while it is still in the womb, and the risk of transmission is much higher during the mother's primary infection. Serious consequences to the fetus include blindness, brain damage, miscarriage, premature delivery, and death. In addition to the problem of infections during the pregnancy, an active lesion in or around the vagina at the time of delivery warrants a cesarean delivery. This is done to decrease the chances of viral exposure and possible infection in the newborn at the time of delivery.

In newborns whose mothers have known active herpes (remember that the total number of cases is unknown because so many women are asymptomatic), only .01 to .1 percent will contract herpes infections. Although the risk of serious fetal infection is extremely small (and even less in recurrent outbreaks than in primary infections), the consequences are potentially catastrophic.

Herpes poses one other medical risk that it shares with other genital infections that produce ulcers. The AIDS virus can enter the body more easily when there are breaks in the skin on or near the genitals. It is very clear that the heterosexual spread of AIDS in Africa has been facilitated by the presence of several STDs, including herpes, which cause open sores and ulcers on the genitals of both men and women. The added risk of HIV transmission only further enforces the need for safer-sex practices everywhere.

Monogamy (with a monogamous partner) is obviously the cornerstone of safer sex. Although condoms protect the vaginal, cervical, and penile mucosa and skin from viral contact, herpes outbreaks frequently occur on the labia, in the skin folds of the groin, on the scrotum, on the buttocks, and at the base of the spine. Female condoms may offer a somewhat larger area of protection than male condoms. Dental dams (the latex shield used during dental work that can be obtained at many women's health clinics) can be used to cover and protect the entire vulva during oral sex or mutual masturbation, but these barrier methods will not provide complete protection from exposure. Abstaining from sex until the sores are healed will offer some protection, but most outbreaks occur without producing symptoms and can be spread during these asymptomatic periods.

Treatment

Medical science has not yet learned how to cure viruses, and herpes is no exception. The herpes virus establishes itself on the genitals and then permanently makes its home in the nerve cells of the spinal cord. Reducing the number of outbreaks depends on maintaining general good health, including good nutrition, proper rest, and stress reduction. Once an outbreak occurs, the infected area should be kept clean and dry in an effort to prevent bacterial infection of the open sores. Do not scratch, squeeze, or rub the blisters, and wash your hands with soap and water immediately if contact does occur. Sexual activity can spread the virus to an uninfected partner and can irritate the skin around the infected area, possibly slowing the healing process. Therefore, sexual relations should be avoided until after the sores crust over.

The only medication that seems to shorten the length of an outbreak and reduce its severity is acyclovir (*Zovirax*). This drug comes in an intravenous form for the most severe infections that require hospitalization and also comes in pill and ointment preparations. The pill form is more effective than the ointment and is the most commonly used treatment for genital herpes. The treatment should be started with the onset of symptoms and continued until the symptoms subside (usually 5 to 10 days). If you suffer from frequent outbreaks, a long-term course (up to 6 months) may be prescribed in order to reduce the number of future outbreaks. Acyclovir may be used by pregnant women; theories about the drug's risk to the fetus have not been proved. Acyclovir may be indicated in severe cases because the virus could be more damaging to the fetus than the unknown risks of the drug.

PELVIC INFLAMMATORY DISEASE (PID)

Pelvic inflammatory disease refers to an infection of the uterus, fallopian tubes, and ovaries that originates in the vagina and cervix and ascends into the upper pelvic organs. Although the initial infective organism is generally either gonorrhea or chlamydia, other bacteria may cause PID. The spread of the infection into the upper pelvic organs usually involves multiple species of bacteria and other organisms that work together to infect the uterus, tubes, and ovaries. The ability of these bacteria to migrate from the vagina into the uterus is thought to come about by the breakdown of the normal protective barrier created by the cervical mucus. Another theory is that sperm may facilitate the upward spread of infection, especially in cases that involve chlamydia. In addition it is thought that infective organisms may travel into the upper pelvic organs more easily during menstruation.

Symptoms

PID affects at least 1 million women a year in the United States. Almost 20 percent of these cases occur in teenagers. These numbers are considered low estimates, since mild PID is usually not treated in hospitals and treatment reporting is not required. In fact, some cases of PID are so mild that they go undetected even though they can cause serious long-term complications.

Severe PID is associated with the symptoms of fever, pelvic pain, vaginal discharge, and sometimes pain up under the rib cage on the right side. Severe PID occurs in two forms: acute and chronic. Acute

PID is a short-term infection that lasts only one to two weeks, and, if immediately and properly treated, it may produce no serious complications. Chronic PID is a long-lasting and usually recurrent form of the disease characterized by repetitive bouts of pelvic pain and signs of pelvic infection. Once bacteria and other organisms establish themselves in the uterus and fallopian tubes, the organs become inflamed, pus forms, and scarring occurs in and around the tubes. As a result, the tubes become deformed and/or defective in their role of transporters of sperm and eggs.

The long-term complications of PID are chronic pelvic pain, infertility, and tubal (ectopic) pregnancy. The disease results in infertility in at least 100,000 women each year, and is thought to be the cause of at least 70,000 ectopic pregnancies annually. There is a six- to tenfold increase in the risk of developing an ectopic pregnancy if a woman has had PID, even if the infection was asymptomatic. Increased long-term complications of pelvic pain, infertility, and ectopic pregnancy can also be expected by women who have had repeated bouts of PID.

Treatment

Treatment depends upon prompt diagnosis with proper blood tests and cervical cultures, a thorough medical history and physical exam, and sometimes even laparoscopy. Antibiotics (usually in combination) that cover a broad range of potentially infective organisms must be taken for at least 10 to 14 days. If the infection is very severe, hospitalization may be required for the administration of intravenous antibiotics. If a woman with PID was wearing an intrauterine device at the time of the infection, it should be removed in most cases. Most health-care professionals feel that the device should not be used by women who have previously had PID, since it is believed that the device may increase the risk of recurrent infection. Male sexual partners of women diagnosed with PID should also be treated with a full course of antibiotics, whether or not they are symptomatic. Even though sexual partners may or may not show signs of infection, they may be harboring the organisms that can cause PID.

Prevention

The prevention of PID is best accomplished by having a monogamous relationship. Condoms are important in protecting against the spread of those organisms that cause PID. Diaphragms and cervical caps with spermicide are also considered helpful in reducing the incidence of infections that cause PID. The female condom is thought to be effective in preventing the spread of these heterosexually transmitted organisms.

SYPHILIS

Syphilis is an infection caused by a coil-shaped bacterial organism (spirochete) called *Treponema pallidum*. The organism is fragile and will die quickly when exposed to heat or air. Thus, it cannot live in towels or on toilet seats. The infection is generally spread during sex when the mucous membranes of the genitals, mouth, or anus of one partner come in contact with the infected genitals of the other. The disease can also be spread if the infected area comes in contact with any open skin (a cut, crack, or blister). In addition, the infection can pass from an infected mother to her fetus, or it may be spread by contaminated blood (as with shared needles during intravenous drug use) or by accidental needle-stick injuries incurred by medical personnel. In the United States, blood transfusions are routinely screened for the presence of syphilis infection.

The incidence of syphilis has fluctuated over the last 50 years. Between 1940 and the late 1950s, the incidence dropped dramatically. But in the early 1960s and again during the 1980s, the incidence of the disease rose sharply and is now the highest it has been since 1950. Although the U.S. Public Health Service requires reporting of the disease, many experts believe that only 1 in 8 cases is actually reported. Even with this gross underestimation, the incidence of the disease in the United States is currently 15 cases per 100,000 people.

Symptoms

The first sign of a syphilis infection is a painless ulcer called a chancre. The chancre, which is the hallmark of primary syphilis, may occur in the mouth, anus, rectum, vagina, on the external genitals, cervix, or tongue, or wherever the site of transmission has occurred. This open sore will usually develop within 2 to 6 weeks (but as early as 10 days and as late as 3 months) from the time of initial exposure to the bacterium. Because the ulcer is painless, it can easily be overlooked. The ulcer is usually seen as a raised ring of red tissue that often produces a clear yellow discharge. However, the lesion of primary syphilis has been called "the great imitator"; because its appearance varies so widely, any genital or skin lesion that does not heal within two weeks should be considered suspicious. It is during the chancre stage that syphilis is most contagious. If left untreated, the chancre will heal in 5 to 8 weeks, but the disease is not over when the ulcer heals. It will then progress to secondary syphilis.

Secondary syphilis is characterized by generalized symptoms such as headache, sore throat, fever, malaise, swollen glands, and a slightly raised red rash that may appear on any part of the body, including the palms of the hands and the soles of the feet. These symptoms may occur anywhere from 2 to 12 weeks after the disappearance of the chancre and may be so mild as to go unnoticed. However, the rash, even a mild one, contains active spirochetes and is contagious. This means that if there is any break in the rash-covered skin, the disease can be easily spread during sexual or even casual contact (like a handshake). Sometimes secondary syphilis is accompanied by broad, flat, slightly raised mucous patches on the mouth and external genitals, in the skin folds of the groin, under the breasts, and around the anus. These are called *condylomata lata*. The signs and symptoms of secondary syphilis usually disappear over the course of several weeks to months, but they can reappear and be contagious episodically over the next one to two years.

If untreated, secondary syphilis will become quiescent and noncontagious. This latent phase may, in some cases, last for the rest of one's life. But in 15 to 40 percent of cases, the disease will progress to the late or tertiary stage. This stage can last for many years and is characterized by systemic damage by the bacteria to any part of the body. The ravages of the disease can result in blindness, brain damage, psychosis, peripheral nerve damage, joint pain and deterioration, heart damage, and an almost endless list of other serious medical problems. In women, tertiary syphilis occasionally produces an ulcerative nodule on the vulva called a *gumma* that can serve as a site of contagious bacteria.

During any stage of untreated syphilis, the disease can be transmitted by a mother to her fetus. The spirochete can pass through the placenta and infect the fetus any time after 16 weeks. In addition, it is thought that syphilis can increase the rate of miscarriage. Infection of the unborn baby can result in various congenital malformations, liver and spleen enlargement with or without jaundice, excess fluid in the skin or abdominal cavity and around the heart, open and contagious skin sores, mental retardation, meningitis, premature delivery, and miscarriages. If treatment is begun during pregnancy, the infection will be cured in both the mother and the fetus, but the fetus will be born with whatever damage the disease has already caused. If left untreated, the fetus will be born with congenital syphilis.

When the initial stages of the disease go unnoticed, diagnosis of syphilis can be difficult. Most developed countries require a blood test for syphilis at the time a couple applies for a marriage license. Most states in the United States require syphilis testing during pregnancy. The two blood-screening tests currently available are the VDRL (venereal disease research laboratory) and the RPR (rapid plasma reagin). These tests are nonspecific and can turn positive in the presence of some viral and autoimmune diseases (such as lupus, Reynaud's disease, or rheumatoid arthritis). They can also be falsely negative in early primary syphilis (up to four weeks after initial exposure and infection), in latent syphilis, and in tertiary syphilis. If the initial screening test is positive or if the patient's medical history in any way indicates that an infection has occurred, then a specific antibody test for the organism, called a treponeme, should be performed. Although antibody tests measure one's immune response products (syphilis-specific antibodies) used to fight the disease, such tests remain positive throughout a person's life and cannot detect a new or recent reinfection. Syphilis, like gonorrhea and chlamydia, can be treated, but previous infection and treatment does not confer any immunity, so reinfection may occur again and again. If a repeat infection is suspected, then a series of blood tests looking for a rise in the rate of antibody response should be performed.

Treatment

Once the diagnosis of syphilis has been made, tests for other STDs should be done and the patient and her partner should be treated. Penicillin remains the best treatment for syphilis, but it must be given as an injection. Certain other high-potency injectable antibiotics can also be used in large doses (they must be given in the buttocks). Tetracycline, doxycycline (*Doryx, Vibramycin*), or erythromycin (*ERYC, E-Mycin*) pills may be less painful alternatives, but they do not effect the same rate of cure and are not ever recommended during pregnancy.

Late latent syphilis, one phase of tertiary syphilis, requires a different type of injectable penicillin that is given for three consecutive weeks. Neurosyphilis is another phase of tertiary syphilis. This is diagnosed when the treponemal infection is isolated from the fluid around the brain or spinal cord. The recommended treatment is yet another penicillin preparation given intravenously every 4 hours for 10 to 14 days. For pregnant women, the treatment of tertiary syphilis is the same. For all stages of syphilis, periodic retesting is necessary to test for a complete cure. For penicillin-allergic patients, there is a complex, difficult process called desensitization, which can supersede the allergy to allow treatment. This is especially crucial during pregnancy, when erythromycin is not considered effective in preventing congenital syphilis.

As with other STDs, the best treatment is prevention, and safer-sex practices are the key. Any ulcerative genital lesion (whether caused by syphilis, herpes, or granuloma inguinale, etc.) increases the ability for the AIDS virus to pass from one partner to another. If you are diagnosed with syphilis, your health-care provider should discuss safer-sex practices with you, and you and your partner should have HIV testing.

TRICHOMONIASIS

Trichomonas vaginalis is a sexually transmissible organism that causes trichomoniasis infection in the lower genitourinary tracts of men and women. It is a protozoan, a single-celled organism with a large body and a tail that allows it to "swim" much as a sperm does. Trichomoniasis (commonly known as "trich") is usually contracted through heterosexual intercourse or vulval contact during lesbian sex. Because a protozoan is a relatively hardy organism, it can also be spread by casual means, including sharing wet towels or wet bathing suits. Sexual play toys and vaginal douche nozzles are other modes of transmission.

Symptoms

Approximately 15 percent of women in their reproductive years are carriers of trichomoniasis, but only one-third of these women exhibit any symptoms. Trich is most common in women with more than one sexual partner. These are most commonly younger women—but it is not limited to any age group. Typically, the most common symptom is vaginal discharge that may be green, yellow, white, or grey; thick, thin, or frothy; and usually malodorous. The infection may be accompanied by vulval or vaginal itching, redness, swelling, or pain, and may cause discomfort during sexual intercourse or urination. The symptoms are often worse just after a menstrual period, and they can be very acute during pregnancy. The incubation period is anywhere from 4 to 28 days. Although the symptoms of trichomoniasis can be uncomfortable and annoying, the infection is not thought to cause any long-term or serious complications.

The diagnosis of trichomoniasis is made by inspecting a drop of the vaginal discharge under a microscope. In most cases, the organisms that cause the disease can be easily seen swimming across the slide, propelled by their whiplike tails.

Trichomoniasis can be treated with antibiotics, and the medication of choice is metronidazole (*Flagyl*) tablets, given as one 2-gram dose. If the infection is not cured, or it returns, then 500-milligram metronidazole tablets will be prescribed two a day for a week for you and your partner. This medication has the same effect as disulfiram (*Antabuse*); it causes vomiting when used with alcohol, so drinking anything alcoholic is contraindicated while on metronidazole. If one partner is diagnosed, then all partners should be treated.

Metronidazole capsules are not recommended for women in their first trimester of pregnancy, and other (usually less effective) treatments are recommended, although they may only relieve the symptoms and not cure the infection. If you are prone to recurrent infections, mild vinegar, medicated douches, or boric acid capsules are helpful in making the vaginal environment less hospitable to the *Trichomonas* organism. However, you should evaluate whether reinfection is occurring from your partner. Although a vaginal gel containing metronidazole is now available, it is not recommended for the treatment of trichomoniasis at this time.

Only 20 percent of infected men show symptoms of an infection. Condoms are effective in preventing the passage of trichomoniasis from male to male or male to female, and they should be used during the entire treatment course of the infection. Sex toys should not be shared by anyone. During lesbian sex, dental dams should be used.

OTHER STDs

There are several other less common STDs, and they are briefly described here.

Chancroid

This disease is characterized by a painful vulval ulcer that is usually accompanied by vulval swelling and, in about half the cases, enlargement of the lymph nodes in the groin. It is caused by the bacterial organism *Hemophilus ducreyi*. Although this STD used to be uncommon in the United States, it has become much more prevalent in the last decade.

Diagnosis is difficult and requires careful removal of the bacterium from under the crust of the ulcer. Expert preparation of a stained slide is necessary so that the organism can be properly identified. Antibiotic treatment with 500 milligrams of oral erythromycin four times a day for seven days, or with a single shot of Ceftriaxone (*Rocephin*) is currently recommended. Ciprofloxacin (*Cipro*) pills (500 milligrams) taken twice a day for three days are an acceptable alternative treatment. Any partner, male or female, who has had sex with someone who develops chancroid within 10 days of that encounter should also be treated. As has been noted in countries where chancroid has been a common STD, the transmission of HIV is facilitated by the presence of any genital ulcer. The female condom offers some protection in the prevention of this and other ulcerative vulval diseases.

Lymphogranuloma Venereum (LGV)

An uncommon STD in the United States, lymphogranuloma venereum is caused by various strains of the *Chlamydia trachomatis* organism. LGV is characterized by the development of a small pustule or ulcer on the vulva or around the anus only a few days after exposure. This lesion disappears quickly and is followed by swelling of the lymph nodes in the groin. The nodes frequently become so infected that they form large abscesses that can drain spontaneously. Treatment requires that all partners take 100 milligrams of doxycycline twice a day for 21 days.

Pubic Lice

Pubic lice, commonly known as "crabs," are easily transmitted during sexual contact between heterosexual, homosexual, or bisexual persons. This hardy parasite, *Pediculosis pubis*, can also be transmitted by contact with infected inanimate objects such as bed sheets, towels, locker room benches, and even toilet seats. This tiny six-legged creature and the eggs (nits) it lays at the base of the pubic hairs can be easily identified with a magnifying glass.

The most common symptom of infestation is itching in the pubic and perianal region. Recommended treatment requires the application of either a preparation of permethrin (1 percent) cream, or pyrethrins and piperonyl butoxide, to all infected areas. These products are insecticides and must be washed off after 10 minutes. Lindane (1 percent) shampoo, applied for four minutes and then washed off completely, is an alternative regimen, but it cannot be used by pregnant or lactating women. Pregnant women may use permethrin, pyrethrins, or piperonyl butoxide. All sexual partners should also be treated. In addition, all clothing, bed linens, and towels should be washed in hot water and dried on the hot cycle; they can also be dry-cleaned instead. If symptoms of pubic lice persist, reevaluation should be done a week after treatment. If nits or lice are still present, retreatment of all affected parties and rewashing of all contaminated articles must be performed. In extreme cases, the pubic area is shaved.

Viral Hepatitis

Viral hepatitis is common among homosexual and bisexual men and their male and female partners. It is also widespread among heterosexual men and women who are not monogamous and among IV drug users and their sexual partners. This virus can be spread through the exchange of blood, semen, vaginal secretions, and feces, and is easier to transmit than the AIDS virus. Most acute cases are totally asymptomatic, but the long-term chronic, active form of the disease can lead to liver cancer and death.

As with most viral diseases, there is no treatment for hepatitis infection. However, a vaccine is available for anyone who is at high risk for contracting the disease (health-care workers, homosexual/ bisexual men and their partners, IV drug users and their sexual partners, and prostitutes). If you have good reason to believe that you have had sex with someone who has been recently diagnosed with hepatitis B (or who is a hepatitis B carrier), then you snould consider getting a shot of hepatitis B immune globulin within 14 days of exposure. This medication helps prevent the virus from establishing itself and thereby infecting the liver. As with other STDs, the spread of viral hepatitis can be reduced by the rigorous practice of safer sex. The vaccine is recommended for people whose jobs put them at risk for hepatitis B. It is not recommended instead of safer sex or discontinuation of IV drug usage, but it will confer immunity for those who continue to put themselves at risk.

11

MENOPAUSE

The word "menopause" is derived from two Greek roots: *Men* means "month" and *pausis* means "stop." The actual significance of menopause is one single event—your last menstrual period. "Perimenopause" is the time just before menopause, when symptoms first start to appear, and it continues up to the postmenopausal period. You have arrived at the postmenopausal time of your life when you have completed a full year without having another period.

Perimenopause may be a matter of only a few years or it may encompass as many as 10 years of a woman's life. In the past, this period was referred to as the "climacteric," literally "rung of the ladder" in Greek. This term is synonymous with perimenopause, but it is rarely used today except in medical texts.

Menopause is not a disease: It is the time when the production of ovarian estrogen begins to wane. With the natural decrease in estrogen production, many symptoms may occur that are easy to identify.

These symptoms do not indicate that something is wrong. The image of menopause must change from the pathological to a natural, normal event of life.

Although the physiology of menopause is constant in women, the symptoms vary from culture to culture. In Japan, for example, the most common complaint of menopause is stiff shoulders. However, in our culture women most commonly complain of hot flashes and mood swings. Menopause is a powerful marker in the aging process. Menopause does mark the end of the reproductive years, but it also marks the beginning of a new and productive phase of your life.

THE PHYSIOLOGY OF MENOPAUSE

As a 20-week fetus in her mother's womb, a human female has present in her ovaries 6 to 7 million eggs. But even in utero, the aging process begins, and by the time a female baby is born, she will have only about 1 to 2 million eggs left. By the time a young girl reaches menarche (the onset of menses) and begins to menstruate, she will have about 300,000 to 400,000 eggs left to mature. During the average woman's reproductive life span, she will produce only 400 to 500 mature eggs capable of being fertilized. The remainder will wither and die.

Because these follicles (immature eggs) are a main source of estrogen production, their atrophy results in lower estrogen production. That means that the ovaries have less and less reproductive potential. After a woman reaches age 35, this process accelerates until the number of follicles is further decreased to the point when ovulation stops completely. This cessation of ovulation correlates with menopause and occurs on the average at about age 51.

The ovaries are not the only place where estrogen is produced. There is a type of estrogen called estrone that is produced by fat cells. Estrone is less potent than ovarian estrogen, but the production from the fat cells is fairly consistent throughout a woman's life. Although estrone production may diminish slightly with age, it does not cease at menopause. For this reason, women with an excess of body fat exhibit fewer menopausal symptoms. Also during this midlife period, the metabolic rate begins to slow down and more calories will be stored as fat. This is a protective phenomenon that allows for some production of estrogen in the later years. It is also the reason that the contours of a woman's body change as she approaches the age of menopause. Therefore, the menopausal state does not mean that there is no estrogen production, but rather that there is a difference in the amount, the production site, and type of estrogen produced.

COMMON SYMPTOMS OF PERIMENOPAUSE

Estrogen receptors are located throughout the body, so the decline in estrogen production has an effect on many organs, including the brain. Many factors influence the degree of discomfort experienced by each woman during perimenopause. These factors include age, the time frame in which the decrease in estrogen occurs, the amount of body fat, the social setting, and a woman's knowledge and interpretation of what is occurring. In addition, because estrogen has a direct effect on brain tissue, many women have vague feelings that affect their sense of well-being, their short-term memory, and their ability to make decisions.

Hot Flashes

A hot flash is the sudden sensation of warmth, usually in the head, neck, and chest. It is a subjective symptom in response to changes in blood vessels and the muscles that surround those vessels (a vasomotor response) and is accompanied by a surge of pituitary LH. A hot flash is accompanied by a rise in the temperature of the skin that produces the sense of warmth, and is followed by a flush caused by dilation of the blood vessels in the skin. The duration of a hot flash varies, but it averages between one and five minutes.

The occurrence of hot flashes is the most common complaint of perimenopause for most American and western European women; 85

percent of these women experience them at some point during peri-menopause. The onset of a hot flash is triggered by a multitude of factors that vary from woman to woman, but that may include alcohol intake, heat, stress, or emotional distress. The exact mechanism that creates a hot flash is not known, but it is speculated that the feedback mechanism of the cyclic hormones estrogen and progesterone stimulates nerve cells in the brain. These cells, which lie close to the temperature-regulating system, trigger the response.

There are various relief measures that can alleviate the symptoms of hot flashes. One reliable treatment is estrogen replacement therapy (ERT). Other purported treatments are unreliable and include ergotamine (*Bellergal-S*), methyldopa (*Aldomet*), danazol (*Danocrine*), clonidine (*Catapres*), progesterone (*Gesterol 50*), and many others. All of these drugs have side effects such as high blood pressure, low blood pressure, mood swings, and weight gain. Hot flashes may be helped in some women through acupuncture, herbal remedies, relaxation therapy, and guided imagery. Many others find they don't need to employ any relief measures at all but choose to live with the hot flashes until they simply go away.

Studies have shown that there is a marked relief of symptoms with the institution of hormone replacement therapy (HRT), a combination of estrogen and progesterone therapy. Although many of these studies have been funded by the pharmaceutical industry, they do show results confirming the advantage of estrogen replacement therapy (ERT) in relieving hot flashes. The first large long-term study on HRT, now in process, is being funded and run by the National Institutes of Health.

Night sweats and insomnia go hand in hand with perimenopause. Hot flashes at night can be subtle, interrupting the phase of sleep that allows you to wake up feeling rested. Sometimes they can be violent, jerking you awake from a sound sleep and drenching you in sweat. Because you are wet, you get chilled. This means you must get up and change, which is obviously disruptive to a good night's sleep. Sleep disturbances of any kind can be very debilitating. They can make you feel run down and worn out; they can also make you feel depressed. If you have had a child, the sleepless nights and worn-out days will remind you of the months of getting up with the baby. Fortunately, night sweats are usually a finite condition that gradually become less disruptive until they disappear.

Night sweats will respond to the same treatment therapies you found effective for daytime hot flashes. Although sleeping medications will enable most women to overcome the sleep disturbances associated with decreasing estrogen levels, many of these are addictive. In addition, many of them cause sedation but do not restore restful sleep. These medications include the often prescribed diazepam (*Valium*), alprazolam (*Xanax*), and flurazepam (*Dalmane*). Women who resort to alcohol or sleeping pills at this point in their lives can easily create a pattern of lifelong drug dependency. This is far more serious than the hot flashes these medications were designed to relieve.

Vaginal Changes

The vagina and labia, which are loaded with estrogen receptors, are extremely sensitive to the decrease in estrogen levels during perimenopause. As the estrogen levels decrease, both the fatty tissue in the labia majora (outer vaginal lips) and the thickness of the vaginal lining decrease as well. The thinning of the vaginal lining may lead to dryness, increased vaginitis, burning, and painful intercourse. Vaginal dryness is also increased by reduced secretions from the glands found in the cervical canal and the entrance to the vagina. Lowered estrogen levels may also cause a thinning of pubic hair. Estrogen replacement therapy in the form of pills, patch, or vaginal cream is very helpful in alleviating vaginal symptoms.

There are commercial over-the-counter preparations that are very effective but don't have the side effects of HRT. *Replens* and *Gynemoistrin,* two preparations that can be inserted vaginally three times a week, work well to keep the vagina moist. These preparations work like skin moisturizers; they contain no hormones but are composed of substances that hold water molecules in the cells of the vaginal lining. Lubricating gels, such as *K-Y* jelly, are best used just before intercourse, as they dry out within 20 minutes or so. Do not use any oil-based product, such as petroleum jelly or baby oil, inside the vagina.

These substances are not absorbed and can make the vagina more prone to infection.

Urinary Changes

The lower third of the bladder and the urethra also have many estrogen receptors. As estrogen levels drop, the tissue tone of these urinary outflow organs weakens, allowing urine to leak out. This commonly leads to symptoms of urinary incontinence or frequency. If you are experiencing these symptoms, ERT can produce some relief. There are also exercises that should be done regularly to tone the pelvic floor, a sling of muscles that support the bladder, rectum, and vagina. Tensing and releasing these muscles, as if you were stopping the flow of urine, improves pelvic support. These are called Kegel exercises, and they will keep the muscles of the pelvic floor in good tone and therefore give you more urinary control. Not only do they prevent bladder, rectal, and vaginal relaxation, but they can also greatly enhance your sex life. The improved vaginal tone gives you more sensory pleasure and control during vaginal penetration.

Decreased Libido

Many factors, not just the depletion in ovarian hormones, contribute to the decrease in the desire for sex among some perimenopausal women. Many psychosocial changes occur at the same time as perimenopause. For example, if you have children, they may be reaching their teenage years or young adulthood. If you did not start your family until later in life, you may still be dealing with toddlers. Either situation will produce differing demands and challenges. At the same time, your parents are aging and may require more time and energy. This is also a time when children may be leaving home and you are faced with a change in the relationship between you and your sexual partner. Perimenopause is a time for reassessing your life, relationship, career, and habits. All these factors affect sexual energy and desire.

Men as well as women experience changes in midlife, although men do not experience the dramatic physical changes unique to women. A decrease in sexual desire occurs in both sexes as part of the aging process. As always, if the desire is shared by both partners, then it is not a problem. But other changes or crises may be going on in your relationship that also affect sexual desire. If you do not have a partner or if your partner is not functional (depressed, impotent, drunk, or ill) or not interested, you may find that your sexual desire will wane. If your partner develops a health problem requiring medication that inhibits his or her sex drive, you may find that he or she seems suddenly uninterested in sex. Your sexual relationship may suddenly demand more honest communication and creativity. Hormone replacement therapy may or may not be helpful in maintaining a healthy sexual relationship, but it is certainly only one factor at a complex time in your life.

Sometimes perimenopausal women experience changes in sexual desire that are due to the physical changes induced by decreased estrogen levels. As stated, the vagina responds dramatically to estrogen depletion, and vaginal penetration can therefore become painful. If sex hurts, it is normal for the desire to diminish. The relief measures stated previously (see "Vaginal Changes," page 175) may be all that is needed to restore the desire for sex.

In addition, as the ovaries age, they produce decreasing amounts of testosterone. (This drop in testosterone is much more gradual than the drop in estrogen. In fact, the ovaries usually produce some amount of testosterone for at least 10 years after menopause.) It is believed that the decrease in testosterone, in conjunction with the drop in estrogen levels, greatly affects women's sexual desire. For this reason, some women who opt for HRT find that a combination of estrogen and low-dose testosterone are necessary to restore their libido.

If the problem is not physical but emotional, therapy or group counseling may be extremely helpful. Women's groups offer a supportive atmosphere, and it always helps to realize that you are not the only one going through this. Solutions may be uncovered by sharing experiences and feelings.

It has been shown that women who remain sexually active throughout perimenopause and into the postmenopausal years sustain a higher level of sexual desire. Frequent sex promotes good vaginal health and maintains desire. You need not wait until passion over-whelms you to have sex. Sometimes sexual relations will trigger desire. Keep a lubricant handy if vaginal dryness is a problem.

Mood Swings

Perimenopause is a time of hormonal surges and plunges. It is the mirror image of puberty and may be just as stormy. The mood swings that marked the onset of the reproductive years recur as your repro-ductive capacity diminishes. Some women experience similar mood swings just before menstruation, when their hormone levels temporar-ily drop. And it is not uncommon to see mood swings, emotional changes, and depression as hormone levels plummet after childbirth. For most women, the hormonal extremes of perimenopause eventu-ally taper off as hormonal levels decline. As this happens, the mood swings taper off and eventually go away. The woman whose peri-menopausal period is relatively brief (less than one year) seems to experience fewer mood swings, according to some studies. It is impor-tant to remember that the symptoms of perimenopause are temporary, although they may last from several months to several years. Hormone replacement therapy has been shown to be effective in reducing mood swings for those women who find such changes intolerable. Exercise helps reduce the intensity of the mood swings. In fact, both estrogen and exercise stimulate the release of endorphins, natural brain chemi-cals that reduce pain and stress. Exercise, therefore, can have the same effect as HRT on mood swings.

Depression

Depression in the perimenopausal years is not uncommon. Although it has been linked to decreased hormonal levels, a causal relationship has not been documented. Depression is often a result of the sleep disturbances brought on by night sweats. If you are not sleeping well, there is a greater chance that your work and life may suffer. This inability to "be yourself," the chronic fatigue, and the perception that you are just not able to keep up can lead to diminished self-esteem and depression. This period also coincides with many life changes that can lead to depression. The care of aging parents, the loss of a beloved parent, the so-called empty-nest syndrome, and the family's changing roles can bring on depression—at least temporarily. Depression is common among men as well as women in this age group, and you may have a spouse or partner who also makes demands and depletes your reserves of energy.

Depression is easier to cope with for those women who can identify a cause. Because menopause coincides with a drop in estrogen, many women experience depressive symptoms not unlike those seen just before menstruation or after the birth of a child. For most women, the depression associated with all three events is temporary; however, in a very small percentage of women, depression associated with steep drops in estrogen may be severe and require medical therapy. Many women see no reason for their depression. They have an overall sense of despondency, but they don't know why. It may be enough of a reassurance to recognize depression as a symptom of perimenopause and to understand that it is a difficult but temporary period of transition.

Skin Changes

Skin changes occur in both men and women as they age. The environmental impact of sun exposure and cigarette smoking can have a devastating effect on the skin, promoting drying and wrinkling at an accelerated rate. A lifelong pattern of a balanced diet, proper hygiene, adequate fluid intake, regular use of sunscreen, and avoidance of cigarette smoke will have the greatest impact on maintaining healthy skin.

Postmenopausal women often have a slight increase in facial hair and dry skin. Those who take estrogen replacement therapy report a reduction of dry skin and the itching that may accompany it. Estrogen, however, has not been documented as a treatment for dry skin. Increased facial hair is a common symptom of menopause, whether you are taking estrogen or not.

Bone Changes

It has been clearly shown that bone density decreases in the postmenopausal years. This condition is known as osteoporosis, and the risk of
developing it depends on age, sex, genetic predisposition, weight, and
race. Although both men and women can develop osteoporosis, white
and Asian women who are slim are at higher risk. Women who produce low levels of estrogen are also at higher risk. They include older
women, women who entered menopause prematurely, women who
have had their ovaries removed, and women who are do not ovulate
(for example, long-distance runners and women with anorexia). Eventually, bone mass may decrease to the point where fractures happen
with a minimum of trauma. A woman has reached her maximum bone
mass by the time she is 35 years old. From then on, the density begins
to diminish until menopause, when the rate of demineralization accelerates. Ultimately, this rate levels off, but it leaves older women predisposed to fractures, particularly of the hip, spine, and wrist. Spinal
fractures cause an overall reduction in height as well as moderate or
severe back pain. Of those women who sustain hip fractures, 15 to 20
percent will die from complications; many more than that suffer some
loss of mobility and independence. Osteoporosis is a serious medical
problem whose consequences cannot be underestimated.

Many factors in addition to hormonal levels affect one's bone
mass. Nutrition and proper exercise play a major role in the preserva-
tion of strong bones. Abuse of tobacco and alcohol may speed the loss
of bone density. Cigarette smoking is the biggest factor in bone loss,
but excessive alcohol consumption can also reduce bone density.
However, caffeine and a diet high in animal fats have not been shown
to decrease calcium in the bone, although this was previously believed
to be true. A healthy lifestyle, which includes good nutrition, regular
exercise, and avoidance of excessive caffeine, alcohol, and cigarettes,
should be a lifelong pattern.

If you have difficulty obtaining adequate calcium from your diet,
you can enhance your intake with calcium supplements. Calcium car-
bonate, calcium lactate, or calcium gluconate will provide adequate
elemental calcium. One thousand mg a day of elemental calcium is

recommended if you are taking estrogen supplementation. If you are young and produce estrogen, 1,000 mg is also recommended. If you are menopausal and not taking estrogen, 1,500 mg is recommended.

However, no calcium supplement is nearly as well absorbed as dietary calcium. Dairy products such as milk, yogurt, and cheese contain large amounts of calcium. Other foods that contain calcium include dark green vegetables, canned fish, and oysters. If you are aware of nutritional or other bad habits as you approach menopause, it is not too late to change them and gain benefit from those changes.

Bone mass can be measured at several sites (the wrist, lower arm, and spine) and by several different techniques (dual energy X-ray absorptiometry or single-photon absorptiometry, to name only two). Although there is no doubt that low bone mass is associated with enormously elevated rates of bone fractures (particularly of the spine), there is no proof that expensive bone tests are reliable. They should not be your sole reason for deciding to increase regular exercise, improve dietary habits, or embark on long-term hormonal or other medical therapies.

Osteoporosis in postmenopausal women is greatly delayed by the use of estrogen. This has been clearly shown in many reliable studies. Estrogen shows its best effect in reducing bone loss if started soon after menopause has begun, and certainly not later than 5 to 10 years thereafter. Estrogen's effectiveness in reducing bone loss continues only for as long as it is being used: Once you stop taking estrogen, bone loss will begin again. However, women should not view estrogen as their only option for healthy bones. A good, nutritious diet that contains adequate amounts of calcium and vitamin D (obtained primarily by exposure to sunlight), coupled with regular exercise, will also greatly retard bone loss. Estrogen plus exercise and a balanced diet will maintain the greatest bone strength. Estrogen replacement therapy alone will not substitute for adequate exercise and a healthy diet high in calcium and vitamin D.

There are other medications that have been suggested for women at high risk for developing osteoporosis who cannot or will not take estrogen. These include etidronate (*Didronel*), calcitonin (*Calcimer*), sodium fluoride, and parathyroid hormone. None of these therapies has been tested for long-term use, and many produce serious side effects like nausea and flushing. Some, like calcitonin (available only by injection), are prohibitively expensive, costing more than $3,500 a year.

Heart Disease

At about the time of menopause, the rate of heart disease in women increases. For postmenopausal women, the death rate from heart disease is more than 10 times the rate from breast cancer. Therefore, the dangers of cardiovascular disease, like breast cancer, must be addressed. There is a large body of evidence showing that women who have low levels of serum cholesterol, with high HDL (high-density lipoprotein, the "good" cholesterol) and a low LDL (low-density lipoprotein, the "bad" cholesterol), are at lower risk of developing heart disease. The road to good cardiovascular health is based on a healthy diet (in which less than 30 percent of your caloric intake comes from dietary fat) and adequate exercise. For postmenopausal women, a great deal has been written about the benefit of estrogen replacement therapy in reducing the risk of cardiovascular disease. Unfortunately, thus far no large-scale study has been performed that was not biased in its selection of subjects. The bias comes from the fact that the studies are done only on women who choose to go on (and stay on) hormone replacement therapy. Many of the women drop out of these studies. Women who choose to use estrogen replacement are a select group who may already have a lower risk of heart disease. Therefore, although it seems that estrogen may indeed reduce the risk of heart disease, there is as yet no proof that it does in the general population.

TREATMENT

Hormone Replacement Therapy

There is a place for the use of estrogen and/or progesterone in the control of symptoms and reduction of long-term health risks associated with menopause. There is no question that estrogen will reduce menopausal symptoms such as hot flashes, night sweats, vaginal dryness, and many of the other symptoms previously described. Some women have tried other options, which they have found inadequate, whereas other women have no interest in trying anything other than hormone replacement therapy (HRT). Hormone replacement is not for everyone. You and your health-care provider must discuss your family and medical history, diet, exercise program, psychosocial situation, and support system before choosing what treatment plan, if any, is best for you.

In addition, estrogen, if taken as a long-term therapy, provides benefits in preventing osteoporosis and possibly heart disease. Since women in America now live on average until age 80, most women will spend one-third of their lives in the postmenopausal period. Many women will opt to take long-term HRT to maintain the health of the vagina and bladder, preserve bone strength, and perhaps prevent heart disease.

Dosage

There are various natural and synthetic estrogen preparations available in the United States. The two most commonly used are conjugated equine estrogen (made from the urine of pregnant mares) and estradiol. Conjugated equine estrogen (*Premarin*) comes in various dosages, and the most frequently prescribed is 0.625 milligram given orally. A higher dose (1.25 mg) may initially be necessary to control hot flashes and other symptoms of perimenopause, but usually the dose can return to 0.625 milligram soon after the symptoms are under control. For long-term use, this level is thought to be the lowest dose that will prevent osteoporosis. Oral estradiol (*Estrace*) is usually prescribed at a dose of 1 milligram daily. Initially, a 1.5- or 2.0-milligram dosage daily may be required to control the symptoms of perimenopause, but this may be lowered to 1 milligram once symptom control is achieved. For long-term use, 1 milligram daily is thought to be the lowest dose that will prevent osteoporosis, although new studies indicate that 0.5 mg may be adequate. In addition, estradiol comes as a skin patch (*Estraderm*). The two dosages available (0.05 mg and 0.1 mg) are equivalent to 0.625 milligram of equine estrogen/1 milligram of oral estradiol and to 1.25 milligrams of equine estradiol/2.0 milligrams of oral estradiol respectively. The patch stays on for 3¹/₂ days and is then removed. A new patch is then applied to a different site. The best sites to apply the patch are the upper outer thigh and the buttocks. (There have been reports about outbreaks of skin rash when the patch is applied to the abdomen.)

Continuous use of ERT will increase your risk ninefold of developing endometrial cancer (cancer of the uterine lining). When this link was first discovered, noncontinuous estrogen therapy was recommended—i.e., taking estrogen for the first 25 days of the month and taking no hormones for the remaining days of the month. This regimen did lower the risk of developing endometrial cancer, but some risk still persisted. It was then discovered that if progesterone was added to the estrogen therapy, the risk of developing uterine cancer would be no greater than that found in the general population.

The hormone schedule that is most often employed has incorporated both of these regimens: daily oral estrogen for the first 25 days of the month with additional progesterone for days 14 through 25. Although some caregivers still use this schedule, it has two drawbacks. First, it leaves you without any estrogen at the end of the month, when hot flashes and other symptoms can occur; second, one schedule composed of different regimens for days 1 through 25 and for days 14 through 25 is not particularly easy to remember, and many women find it confusing. Today most caregivers who recommend cyclic estrogen and progesterone suggest that the estrogen be taken daily and that the progesterone be taken the first 12 or 13 days of the calendar month.

The type of progesterone used in the United States is most frequently medroxyprogesterone acetate (*Provera*), and the most common dose is 5 milligrams. (The second most popular form of progesterone is norethindrone [*Micronor*] with an equivalent dose of 2.5 mg.) If the estrogen patch is being used, it is prescribed exactly twice a week (e.g., Wednesday night and Sunday morning), again with the progesterone for the first 12 or 13 days of the month. If you no longer have a uterus, you don't have to worry about the risks of uterine cancer and need not take any progesterone in conjunction with your estrogen.

Although the progesterone will protect your uterine lining from cancer, it has several drawbacks. Its side effects include bloating, mood swings, weight gain, breast tenderness, and, each month while you stop taking it, a certain amount of bleeding. For some women, particularly when they first start taking HRT, the bleeding may be heavy— as heavy as, or even heavier than, a normal period. This monthly bleeding will usually diminish, and after many years it may entirely disappear. In an effort to reduce the premenstrual-like symptoms associated with progesterone, and to stop the monthly bleeding associated with its cyclic use, a lower dose of progesterone (2.5 mg of medroxyprogesterone or 1.0 mg of norethindrone) may be taken daily. If you take both hormones every day, over the long term you can expect a cessation of all menseslike bleeding. Unfortunately, the long term is quite long for some women. Continuous combined therapy may cause irregular and unpredictable bleeding for the first 3, 6, and even 12 months of use. If you can tolerate this adjustment period, you can then expect no bleeding at all.

Risks and Benefits

How do you decide if hormone replacement therapy will benefit you? Why are you interested in HRT? For the relief it offers for the symptoms of perimenopause, or for the long-term protection it offers your bones and possibly your heart? What other measures could you try or have you tried? What is your weight? If you are obese, your fat cells are producing estrogen. Therefore, you may still take estrogen, but the risks of uterine cancer increase in obese women with or without estrogen therapy. Also, obesity increases the risk of heart disease with or without ERT. You and your caregiver must make up a list of the pros and cons of HRT that takes into account your particular circumstances.

When should you absolutely not take estrogen? If you have had a stroke, a recent heart attack, a recent history of deep thrombophlebitis or pulmonary embolism, an estrogen-sensitive (dependent) breast cancer, or a recent or advanced uterine cancer, you should *not* consider HRT. If you have a history of recent gallbladder or liver disease, you should not take oral estrogen, because it goes first to the liver and then the gallbladder after being absorbed into the gastrointestinal tract. However, estrogen patches may be a possible alternative, since skin absorption allows the estrogen to bypass the liver initially.

What are the relative drawbacks of estrogen? Clearly, the most controversial at this time is the possible increase in the risk of breast cancer. Although some very large studies seem to show an increased risk of as much as 20 to 30 percent, there are still no definitive studies showing that estrogen actually causes breast cancer. Should you take estrogen if you have a family history of breast cancer? You and your caregiver will have to weigh this against other factors such as osteoporosis and heart disease. If you have had a close female relative with uterine cancer, you may again have some hesitation in taking estrogen. Despite the protective effect of progesterone on the uterine lining, you and your health-care provider must consider whether the benefit that estrogen may provide is worth the potential anxiety and risk it may pose.

Estrogen, particularly in combination with progesterone, can cause several unpleasant side effects, but they are not dangerous. These include breast tenderness, which most women can tolerate by reducing the amount of caffeine they ingest or by taking vitamin E (400 mg. daily); weight gain (which can range from about 5 to 10 pounds); and premenstrual-like symptoms that can sometimes be reduced with a change in the dosage schedule. HRT may occasionally produce irregular bleeding, which requires investigation. Your caregiver may choose to perform a uterine biopsy, which is a rather uncomfortable office procedure, or a D&C, which is an outpatient surgical procedure. Both involve a visit to your caregiver as well as some time and expense.

Estrogen may make you feel better. Although there are only a few studies that look at the effect of estrogen on mood and outlook on life, many women report having more energy and greater concentration, and a feeling of well-being. Estrogen does offer symptomatic relief from hot flashes, vaginal dryness, and night sweats. This symptomatic relief may lead to this greater sense of well-being. Perhaps the studies that have only recently been undertaken will help answer some of these questions.

Obviously, the choice of taking HRT is a complex one. You and your caregiver must do a thorough evaluation of your individual needs before making the decision. Remember that HRT may or may not improve your personal quality of life, but it surely cannot substitute for a healthful lifestyle.

Nonhormonal Treatment

Many women who are affected by menopausal discomforts choose not to use hormonal replacement therapy. Some find relief from various nonhormonal remedies. These include herbal preparations such as sage tea or capsules, evening primrose oil capsules, chickweed, or motherwort. In addition, vitamin E offers relief to some women. As previously mentioned, acupuncture, acupressure, massage therapy, and biofeedback are alternatives that may be explored.

12

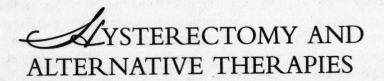# HYSTERECTOMY AND ALTERNATIVE THERAPIES

HYSTERECTOMY

Hysterectomy is the surgical removal of the uterus. *Hystera* is the Greek word for "womb" (*uterus* is the Latin word). The ancient Greeks felt that a woman's emotions were located in her womb, and hysteria in women was attributed to that organ.

In the United States, more than one-third of all women will have had a hysterectomy by age 60. In the late 1970s, hysterectomy was the most common major surgical procedure performed in this country. The peak year was 1978, with 800,000 hysterectomies. Since then, the number of hysterectomies has declined somewhat, in part because of the availability of alternative therapies, and also because of the peer review in major medical centers, which ensures a medical rationale for surgery. However, the number of hysterectomies performed varies greatly in different areas of the country. The highest rate has been in the southeastern United States, where hysterectomy was traditionally used as a form of birth control. This practice is not acceptable today.

The increased focus of the media on female surgery have made women better informed consumers of health care. They have questioned the rationale for surgery and sought alternatives. There are some appropriate indications for hysterectomy, such as life-threatening situations of cancer or hemorrhage, but they constitute only 10 to 12 percent of the cases in which hysterectomy is performed. What about the other 88 to 90 percent? Are they all "unnecessary," as some magazine and newspaper articles say? Major surgery such as hysterectomy *should* have a clear-cut purpose: It should be done to save lives, reduce suffering, or correct physical abnormalities. When hysterectomy is performed to save lives, the purpose is quite clear, as with cancer or other diseases. But who is to say what "suffering" is to any woman? Some woman may tolerate certain symptoms for many years, whereas others may not. In addition, many women "suffer" when they can no longer bear children. So in the case of hysterectomy, relief from suffering is not synonymous with relief from symptoms. For this reason, it is difficult to enumerate specific indications for all hysterectomies.

But if hysterectomy is used as a first step in a problem-solving process, in many cases it is unnecessary surgery. For many conditions, alternative treatments are very effective in relieving symptoms that may otherwise lead to a hysterectomy. For some women, these alternatives are either not attractive or not effective. Much depends on the individual woman, her lifestyle, age, and support system. There are women who do opt for hysterectomy as a first step in order to "get it all over with." This is certainly acceptable if it is the woman's own choice, but it should never be presented as the only choice.

Types

A total hysterectomy refers to the removal of the uterus and cervix. A total hysterectomy, bilateral salpingo-oophorectomy, refers to the removal of the uterus, cervix, fallopian tubes, and ovaries. These procedures may be done through an incision in the abdomen, and are referred to as an abdominal hysterectomy. They may also be done through an incision in the vagina, known as a vaginal hysterectomy.

A newer procedure that allows for the removal of the uterus and the ovaries is the laparoscopically assisted vaginal hysterectomy (LAVH). In most cases of vaginal hysterectomy, it is technically difficult to remove the ovaries. By beginning the procedure with a laparoscope, the ovaries can be removed along with the uterus and cervix. There is another procedure known as a radical hysterectomy that is performed for the treatment of invasive cervical cancer. In this procedure, the uterus, fallopian tubes, and ovaries are removed with a very wide cuff of extra tissue. In extremely rare instances, the uterus alone is removed without removing the cervix. This procedure is called a subtotal or partial hysterectomy. It is usually performed only in emergency situations, when the further operating time necessary to remove the cervix would endanger the patient's life.

ALTERNATIVE THERAPIES

For many years, women were herded into the operating room without fully understanding why and without knowing they had choices. Hysterectomy is often performed not to cure a disease but rather to solve a problem. However, recent developments mean that the problem may respond to newer treatments. Alternative treatments may work quickly and work well. Hysterectomy should not be performed to ease some symptom (like pain and/or bleeding) unless the cause for that symptom has been determined. Before resorting to major surgery, many other relief measures and treatments may be employed. Medications, D&C, laparoscopy, and hysteroscopy are all possible alternatives to hysterectomy, and you may want to consider them before resorting to major surgery.

Women who have suffered for years with painful cycles may go to their health-care providers with hysterectomy as a clear-cut goal. They are tired of the pain and discomfort, and feel that just getting rid of the uterus will make it all go away. It is irresponsible of any health-care practitioner to provide this surgery without counseling about alternatives.

Making the Decision

The decision about hysterectomy is dependent on many factors: a woman's age, whether she has fulfilled any or all of her childbearing plans, approximately how many more menstruating years are in her future, and how well she can physically and mentally tolerate the conditions that made her seek a hysterectomy. For example, bleeding (with or without pain) may become so intense and unpredictable that a woman may stop going out to dinner or might decide not to take a vacation. If you find that your life is revolving around your uterus, then removal of that organ should be one, but not necessarily the first, of your treatment options.

The critical issue to be addressed, especially for young women, is the desire for children. Many women may have talked themselves out of having children so they could relieve their monthly agony. An appropriate treatment plan can be devised to best care for women in this situation. If a woman wants to preserve her fertility, she must pursue alternatives to hysterectomy unless she faces a life-threatening situation. The plan must be agreed to by the woman, her partner, and her doctor. They must weigh all the risks and benefits, costs and time involved, and make the decision together.

ABSOLUTE INDICATIONS FOR HYSTERECTOMY

There are some very real and clear indications for removal of the uterus; others are valid but less absolute. You should never undergo a hysterectomy or, for that matter, any major surgery unless you fully understand why your care provider has proposed it and what, if any, alternatives exist.

The three absolute indications for hysterectomy involve life-threatening conditions: cancer, uncontrollable hemorrhage, or severe infection or rupture of the uterus.

Cancer

Hysterectomy is clearly indicated in the treatment of most cases of uterine, cervical, and ovarian cancer unless the disease is so far advanced that surgery would not significantly prolong or improve life. In advanced cases, chemotherapy and/or radiation therapy may be the preferred treatment if any treatment is chosen at all. If cancer from another organ has spread to the uterus or ovaries, then hysterectomy and removal of the ovaries (oophorectomy) are also indicated.

Hemorrhage

If a woman is bleeding uncontrollably from the uterus (which can happen after a vaginal or cesarean birth) and all other means of stopping the hemorrhage have failed, then hysterectomy is a clearly indicated surgical procedure.

Infection or Rupture

If the uterus, fallopian tubes, and ovaries are overwhelmed by infection that does not respond to antibiotics, the only treatment to save the woman's life is hysterectomy. This is also true if the uterus ruptures during childbirth.

RELATIVE INDICATIONS FOR HYSTERECTOMY

Apart from the conditions mentioned above, the two most common symptoms that lead a woman to hysterectomy are bleeding and pain. Certain pelvic diseases and conditions cause pain, pelvic pressure, and/ or bleeding, and these are described in the following sections. If symptoms cannot be controlled with alternatives, a hysterectomy may be the final step.

Bleeding

Hormone imbalance. Excessive or irregular bleeding may occur at any time during the childbearing years. It is particularly common at the onset of menarche and in perimenopause (those years preceding the actual cessation of menses). Abnormal bleeding in young girls almost always reflects irregular production of hormones in a system that is just getting started, and it usually responds to some combination of hormones. Excessive and/or irregular bleeding in perimenopause may have multiple causes. For example, bleeding may be the result of irregular ovarian hormone production. As the production of eggs diminishes, the ovaries produce estrogen and progesterone in uneven spurts, rather than in the cyclic waves of the earlier reproductive years. These hormone bursts do not allow for the controlled monthly shedding of the uterine lining at the time of menses. Usually, some amount of estrogen is being produced but not enough to trigger the progesterone that in turn triggers menstrual flow. This irregular bleeding normally responds to progesterone therapy or to a combination of estrogen and progesterone.

If the bleeding again becomes excessive during this hormonal therapy, the uterine lining may be evaluated by inserting a hysteroscope through the cervix and into the uterine cavity. If the uterine lining seems normal in appearance, sometimes a dilation and curettage may, for unknown reasons, control the bleeding. During the D&C, cells are obtained that can be sent to a pathologist for a definitive diagnosis.

If bleeding cannot be controlled with hormonal manipulation and/or a D&C, there are some new treatment modalities that may be considered. Gn-RH (gonadotropin-releasing hormone) analogs are a new group of drugs that induce a menopause-like state. They shut off the ovaries' production of female hormones, thereby ending a woman's cycles. If a woman has nearly reached her natural menopause, these drugs may be all that is necessary to induce the inevitable low

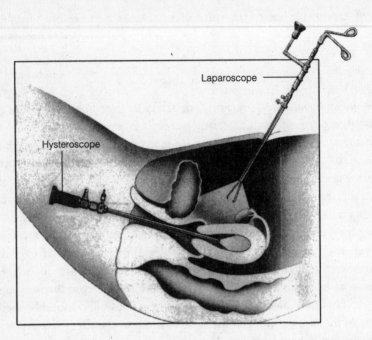

Laparoscope

Hysteroscope

Figure 12.1. Uterine exam using the hysteroscope (shown here with concomitant laparoscopy)

levels of female hormones experienced in menopause. Whether menopause is reached naturally or is artificially induced, it is accompanied by cessation of bleeding and a shrinking of the uterus. It may sound absurd to take a medication (and a very expensive one at that) that will bring on hot flashes, mood swings, and vaginal dryness. But if you are only hastening a natural process ever so slightly, and in so doing are able to avoid major surgery, then the trade-off may be worthwhile for you.

For younger perimenopausal women with excessive uterine bleeding, Gn-RH analogs can be used as a preoperative medication (to prepare the uterus for procedures like uterine ablation). In the past, if the bleeding could not be controlled with D&C or hormonal medications, then the only alternative was an abdominal hysterectomy. Today, Gn-RH gives a woman one more option. If a woman has not yet approached menopause, Gn-RH analogs can be used to temporarily induce a menopausal state, which will cause the uterine lining to atrophy. Gn-RH is used to prepare the uterus for a surgical procedure that is less extensive than an abdominal hysterectomy. Once the uterus is prepared, it may be removed vaginally, or a less invasive procedure can be employed. In some women, the uterine lining may be burned off (ablated) with either electrocautery or laser. This procedure can be performed in a one-day outpatient setting, and routine activities can be resumed in a few days. Approximately 70 to 80 percent of women who undergo this procedure have either no menses or lighter menses. Approximately 10 to 20 percent of women resume normal menstrual flow after uterine ablation, and approximately 10 percent continue to have excessive bleeding that almost always requires hysterectomy.

Besides the uncomfortable nuisance caused by irregular uterine bleeding, women who are losing large amounts of blood every month may become anemic. If an iron-rich diet and iron supplements cannot replenish the blood supply as fast as it is being lost through the uterus, then medical or surgical intervention is necessary.

Fibroids.   Fibroids are benign uterine growths commonly found in more than half of the female population. Whereas many women have fibroids and never experience symptoms, these growths may cause excessive pain and bleeding in some women. When symptoms exist, fibroids should be evaluated for their size and location. This can normally be done by a pelvic exam and/or ultrasound. Fibroids are usually multiple growths and can range in size from a grain of rice to a large grapefruit. They can be located anywhere in the uterus. Some can bulge from the outer surface into the abdominal cavity or hang by a stalk from the outer surface into the cavity. They can form on the inner lining of the uterus and likewise may bulge or hang into the uterine cavity.

If fibroids are small and close to the surface of the uterine lining (a rare occurrence), they can be removed with a hysteroscope inserted through the cervix into the uterus. The uterine cavity is first evaluated. Then, with special tools (like electrocautery, laser, and specially designed miniature surgical instruments), surgical removal of small fib-

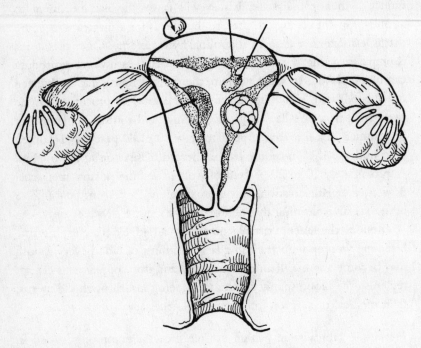

Figure 12.2 Fibroid Tumors

roids and other superficial growths can be accomplished. It is a surgical procedure with a short recuperation time of a day or two.

For women who still want to bear children, myomectomy—the surgical removal of fibroids—can be performed. This is a major surgical procedure, but it allows a woman to retain her childbearing potential. Unfortunately, because only the visible fibroids are removed, microscopic seeds of future fibroids can be left behind. If future childbearing is not a factor and surgery must be preformed, then myomectomy is a poor choice. The fibroids may grow back and symptoms may recur, which would then necessitate additional surgery.

Pelvic pain or pressure.   Pain and/or pelvic pressure are two common symptoms that can lead to hysterectomy. Because these symptoms are very subjective, it is difficult to determine if a hysterectomy is a truly necessary procedure. The health-care provider must assess the pain threshold of the individual. It is obvious that hysterectomy is not the first step in the treatment of pelvic pain. The caregiver should ascertain the cause of the pain to see if it responds to simple medical treatments (like mild pain relievers or oral contraceptive pills) or to nontraditional treatments (like biofeedback, acupuncture, or acupressure). Sometimes excessive bleeding accompanies the pain, making its treatment more complicated.

In evaluating how to approach the treatment of pelvic pain (with or without the presence of bleeding), it is important to evaluate how many more menstruating years are likely. If menopause is approaching within a year or two, it may be possible to tolerate medical treatments until menopause puts an end to the pain or bleeding. If any future childbearing is contemplated, however, this must be factored into the plan before any specific medical or surgical treatment is chosen.

Endometriosis. Endometriosis is a condition in which uterine lining cells (endometrial cells) are found in locations where they don't belong—on the bladder or bowel, behind the uterus, inside the ovary, or almost anywhere else in the body. No matter where these cells are located, they respond to normal cyclic female hormones. When the lining cells are correctly located, they build up with blood during the menstrual cycle and are eventually shed, resulting in menstrual flow. If the cells are located at sites other than the lining of the uterus, they too will build up with blood, but at the end of the cycle the blood will have nowhere to go and will irritate the surrounding tissue. This causes pain the way the trapped blood of a black-and-blue mark causes pain until it is finally absorbed. The pain caused by endometriosis is usually greatest just before and during menses. During the rest of the cycle, much of this microscopic blood is absorbed, but it will reform and be released during the following cycle. For some unknown reason, the size or number of these blood-filled cells does not determine the level of pain a woman experiences. Sometimes one or two freckle-like endometrial cells can cause severe pain, whereas blood-filled ovarian cysts the size of golf balls may cause no pain at all.

If a woman suffers from recurrent cyclic pain that does not respond to pain relievers and/or birth control pills, then endometriosis may be the cause. To diagnose this condition, a laparoscopy should be performed. This is a surgical procedure performed under general anesthesia. A small incision is made just underneath the navel, and a laparoscope is inserted; this allows a look into the abdominal cavity. One or more smaller incisions may be made just above the pubic hair if other instruments are required. This is a simple operation that does not require an overnight stay in the hospital. Most women will be uncomfortable enough afterward to need two or three days to recover, but laparoscopy is not considered major surgery.

If endometriosis is found during laparoscopy, it can be treated with a laser, electrocautery, or other laparoscopic tools. Because implanted cells on surface areas may not be the only sites of the disease, postoperative medication is usually recommended. There are rare cases in which the endometriosis is so severe that much of it cannot be treated through the laparoscope. In these cases, medicines that suppress the production of ovarian estrogen (upon which these implanted cells are dependent) can sometimes shrink the remaining endometriotic cells. The drugs used are birth control pills, danazol (*Danocrine,* which was released in 1976), and Gn-RH analogs (which were approved for the treatment of endometriosis in the late 1980s). When the birth control pill is used in this treatment, it is taken continuously (without any break) for six to nine months. Danazol and Gn-RH analogs are also used for six- to nine-month treatment courses. Both drugs suppress ovarian function, causing a menopause-like state. Danazol resembles Gn-RH analogs in its creation of a pseudomenopause, but in addition to the menopausal side effects like hot flashes, night sweats, and depression common to both drugs, danazol has side effects associated with male hormones. These include acne, weight gain, and increased facial hair.

For infertile women who desire a pregnancy, the end of their treatment course is the optimal time to conceive. If they are successful, their endometriosis often regresses after the delivery of a baby. For other women, the end of the treatment course may offer a pain-free interval of a few months to a few years. These women will often undergo several cycles of surgical and medical management. If the pain cannot be controlled, the treatment of last resort is a hysterectomy with removal of both ovaries. The ovaries are removed because the monthly stimulation of endometriosis is dependent upon ovarian estrogen. Removal of the ovaries, however, is an extreme surgical treatment that should not be done hastily. For those women who have suffered through many years of pain, undertaken trials of unpleasant and expensive drugs, and undergone multiple small surgical procedures, hysterectomy may not only be a last resort; it may also be a godsend.

Adhesions. Other causes of pelvic pain that can be diagnosed and usually treated at the time of laparoscopy include ovarian cysts and pelvic adhesions. Adhesions are internal scars that form during the healing process from previous abdominal or pelvic surgery. They may also result from earlier STDs or from infections resulting from miscarriage, abortion, or childbirth. The treatment for adhesions that are causing intolerable pain is surgery. They can be cut during a laparoscopic procedure that uses laser, electrocautery or other tools. But because adhesions are formed during the healing process, there is no guarantee that they will not reform as the body heals from this invasive procedure.

Major abdominal surgery such as hysterectomy may cause even more internal scarring. Since the scars may involve the intestine and other internal organs, hysterectomy may not help in any way to reduce the pain caused by the adhesions. It may even increase the number and severity of the internal adhesions and therefore cause increased pain. For this reason, major surgery is not usually recommended to treat adhesion-induced pain. Acupuncture or massage therapy is sometimes advised instead.

Sudden uterine growth. Sudden uterine growth can be considered a reason to remove the uterus. Although more than 99.9 percent of uterine fibroids are benign, one related growth is not. This is a leiomyosarcoma, which looks and feels like a benign fibroid but is cancerous. Fibroids don't start out benign and turn into these malignant growths; they begin as fibroids and remain that way. Fibroids and leiomyosarcomas look almost identical on ultrasound, CAT scan, and MRI studies, and they feel the same on pelvic exam. But one identifying feature of the rare cancerous tumor is rapid growth. Since some benign fibroids can also exhibit rapid growth, many doctors believe that all uteri that undergo sudden rapid growth should be removed. Therefore, it is very doubtful that a case of leiomyosarcoma would be mistaken for a benign fibroid and left untreated, since surgery would be indicated.

Uterine prolapse. Uterine prolapse is a condition that can occur at any age but is more commonly seen in older women. Prolapse occurs when the uterus's support structures begin to sag, allowing the uterus to drop through the pelvis and into the vagina. In its most extreme form, complete uterine prolapse, the uterus can actually protrude from the vagina.

Various medical problems are associated with this condition, depending upon the degree of prolapse. If the uterus pulls down the bladder in its path of descent, the woman will have problems holding urine or fully emptying her bladder. If the support system behind the uterus fails, the rectum may pouch out on the underside of the vagina, making complete emptying of the rectum difficult. With the uterus, bladder, and rectum occupying some or all of the vaginal space, intercourse and other sexual activities can be extremely difficult, if not impossible. If the cervix protrudes through the vaginal opening, it can become abraded, sore, and infected.

For these reasons, most women seek relief of this condition. In some cases, the uterus can be pushed back into approximately its original position with the use of a pessary. This is a plastic or hard-rubber device that comes in many sizes and shapes, and is fitted into the vagina, where it can be left in place for up to three months before being removed, cleaned, and replaced by your health-care provider.

In the case of uterine prolapse, hysterectomy is usually recommended for women who cannot be properly fitted with a pessary, who find the pessary unbearable, or who want to remain sexually active but cannot tolerate the type of pessary that allows vaginal penetration during intercourse. Vaginal hysterectomy is usually the preferred procedure, since the weakened support structures allow the surgery to be accomplished easily from the vaginal approach.

Other Choices

Bleeding, pain, and uterine prolapse are conditions that in some cases can be aptly treated with hysterectomy. There are other circumstances in which hysterectomy can be considered a treatment option even though less invasive treatment exists. For instance, if you have a severely abnormal Pap smear and the appropriate workup is performed, you may be told that you have carcinoma *in situ* of the cervix. This is a precancerous condition and can be treated by simply removing a cone-shaped portion of the cervix. After the cone biopsy, you must follow up with frequent Pap smears so that a possible recurrence of the condition is not missed. If a recurrence is not detected early, you will be at risk for developing cancer of the cervix. If you have a family history of cervical cancer, you may find it too frightening to live with that small but potential risk of recurrence. For you, the more invasive procedure of hysterectomy may be called for. Discuss your particular situation with your health-care provider. Except in cases of invasive cancers or in emergencies such as uterine rupture or hemorrhage, most hysterectomies are elective. You should feel comfortable discussing and understanding all other treatment options before deciding on hysterectomy as your best treatment choice.

Recuperation and Risks of a Hysterectomy

Don't let anyone mislead you: Hysterectomy is major surgery. If it is performed through an abdominal incision, expect a hospital stay of 3 or 4 days. If the procedure is performed vaginally, expect a hospital stay of 2 or 3 days. If your particular case requires additional procedures (e.g., suspending the bladder if it has dropped) or if there are unforeseen surgical complications, your stay may be even longer. All major surgical procedures pose the risk of excessive blood loss and could require a transfusion. There are also risks posed by the use of general, spinal, or epidural anesthesia. Infection, which is usually treated with antibiotics, is also a potential risk. Breakdown of the wound can require days or weeks of care by trained family members or by a visiting nurse. This breakdown occurs when there is an infection of skin and underlying layers of tissue, which causes the wound to open. Healing is then a very slow process from the inside out.

Although all of these risks are uncommon, they must be considered whenever hysterectomy is the proposed plan of treatment. You can expect to be unable to perform your normal daily tasks for approximately four to six weeks after abdominal hysterectomy. The postoperative recuperation time after vaginal hysterectomy is between two to four weeks. But after any type of hysterectomy, it may take many more weeks to fully regain your usual level of energy.

Hormones After Hysterectomy

In the past there were surgeons who believed that retaining one ovary during a hysterectomy would halve a woman's risk of later developing ovarian cancer. There is absolutely no factual basis for this belief. If you decide to have a hysterectomy and wish to keep your ovaries, you should keep them both. Unless one ovary appears abnormal, or it is technically difficult to remove the uterus without removing one of the ovaries, there is no logical reason to remove only one ovary.

If you are premenopausal and your ovaries are still producing estrogen, they need not be removed during a hysterectomy. If you are within a few years of menopause, removal of the ovaries is an option to prevent the small risk of ovarian cancer, but you should make this decision with your partner and your physician before the surgery. If you choose to have your ovaries removed—or if they must be removed at the time of the procedure—estrogen replacement therapy (ERT) is recommended for at least the first six postoperative weeks, unless you have an estrogen-dependent cancer that precludes any use of the hormone. When the ovaries are surgically removed, the sudden plunge in estrogen levels may cause severe hot flashes, night sweats, and other menopausal symptoms. Whether or not you wish to embark on long-term ERT, the immediate postoperative period should include estrogen by pill or patch so that estrogen levels are not allowed to suddenly plummet. If you do not wish to remain on estrogen, you can be weaned from it after the six-week course.

If the ovaries are not removed at the time of a hysterectomy, the blood supply to both of them may be interrupted by the surgical procedure itself. In 15 to 25 percent of women who retain their ovaries, ovarian function never fully returns, and such patients will experience menopausal symptoms after surgery. For some women, the disruption of the blood supply is only temporary, and only a brief period of menopausal symptoms is sustained. These women will still undergo menopause at the same age they normally would have.

Emotional Response

The emotional impact of a hysterectomy depends on a multitude of factors. Obviously, if the procedure is being performed as a treatment for cancer, a woman's postoperative emotional state will differ from that of a woman who is freed from uterine prolapse. But a lot depends on one's emotional preparation, no matter what the preoperative diagnosis.

Many cultural differences can influence how people view women who have lost their reproductive organs. Many women consider their womb to be the center of their womanhood. Before you consider undergoing a hysterectomy, you and your sexual partner should discuss what the loss of the uterus will mean to you. For some women, the freedom from long-standing symptoms of bleeding and/or pain may be such a relief that their sex lives are enormously enhanced. For others, having sex after the removal of the uterus feels no different than it did before the surgery. For still other women, hysterectomy may result in a big change in sexual functioning.

For women who lose ovarian function because of the surgery, there may be a decrease in sexual interest because of the drop in ovarian hormones. The loss of libido can be treated with estrogen replacement therapy, but this is not successful for all women. The ovary produces many hormones, not just estrogen. For some women, a program of ERT that doesn't take into account the small quantity of testosterone normally made by the ovaries is just not enough to restore libido. There are a few estrogen/testosterone combinations available, and they are helpful for some women. In the past, these preparations produced unpleasant side effects such as an increase in facial hair and acne. Currently, however, lower doses are available that reduce the unpleasant side effects and help restore libido.

Questions to Ask Your Health-Care Provider

1. Will a hysterectomy resolve my symptoms?
2. Are my symptoms abnormal? If I wait, will they go away or get worse?
3. Is a hysterectomy necessary to cure my condition?
4. What alternative therapies will cure my symptoms?
5. Are the other treatments worth it, or will I end up with a hysterectomy anyway?
6. Will my sexual response be the same?
7. Will my symptoms resolve after menopause?
8. What is the cost?

Getting a Second Opinion

Many insurance companies now require a second opinion before consenting to pay for major surgery. Even if this is not a requirement of your particular insurance company, you may want to consult another health-care provider before deciding on a hysterectomy. Simply make an appointment with a provider and specify that it is for a second opinion. The exam should include a full medical history, a full physical exam, and an evaluation of alternatives to surgery. Sometimes your own physician may give you names to call for a second opinion, but you need not use those people. In small communities where the medical thinking may be less diverse, finding your own second opinion is probably wise. Ask for references from women in the community or call the local hospital. You may also call the public health office for names of physicians, the visiting-nurse association, or the regional medical society. If there is a women's health center in your area, that is also a good place to call for a reference.

13

CANCER RISKS

All cancers are life-altering. Gynecologic cancers affect not only a woman's outlook on life, but also how she views herself sexually. Some women find it difficult to regain their sexual feelings, whether they have a partner or not. If you do have a spouse or partner, open communication and a supportive relationship help ease the pain. This crisis can be a test of a couple's relationship. Individual or couple's counseling may be helpful for some. The most important thing to do is to express your grief, to acknowledge your feelings of loss, and move on from there.

BREAST CANCER

Breast cancer is a disease that touches every woman's life, affecting her, a family member, or a friend. Some medical studies have reported incomplete or inaccurate information to the public. These reports lead to confusion, and sometimes many women will not receive appropriate cancer screening. In addition, many women become so paralyzed with fear of the disease that they avoid screenings that are readily available.

Incidence

The incidence of breast cancer is rising and varies greatly among different races and cultures, but it is more common in Western industrialized societies. The disease is rarely found in men, with only about 600 cases a year being reported. Current statistics from the American Cancer Society indicate that one in eight women will develop cancer of the breast in her lifetime. The rate of incidence increases for women who are in a higher socioeconomic class, women who have never given birth, women who have a late first pregnancy, and women who have a family history of the disease. There are currently 2.4 million women in the United States with breast cancer. In 1994, there were 186,000 new cases. Breast cancer is now the second most common cause of cancer death in women, and 48,000 women die annually from the disease. Recently, lung cancer surpassed breast cancer as the number-one cause of cancer death in women.

Risk Factors

The most important risk factor in developing breast cancer is being a woman. Currently the cause of breast cancer is still unknown. Several studies have indicated possible risk factors, but none of these studies has been conclusive. Among the many factors that have been implicated are dietary fats, alcohol, caffeine, deodorants, oral contraceptive pills, and hormone replacement therapy. Many of these factors have been part of women's lives for centuries, even millennia. Alcohol has been found in Egyptian tombs, caffeine has been part of the Western diet for centuries, and red meat has been a dietary staple in most cultures since prehistoric times. What has changed is what we feed our farm animals, the air we breathe, the water we drink, and the radiation to which we are exposed. It is therefore possible that the greatly increased incidence of breast cancer is due to environmental factors.

Women with fibrocystic breasts were formerly thought to be at higher risk for breast cancer, but several studies have shown that this cannot be substantiated. Women with first-degree relatives (mothers, sisters, or daughters) who had breast cancer are at a substantially higher risk of getting the disease, especially if the family member had breast cancer before menopause. It must be noted, however, that 70 percent of women with breast cancer have no family history of the disease. Breast cancer is more common as women get older, but the older woman with breast cancer has a better prognosis for long-term survival.

There are several other groups of women who have shown a higher incidence of the disease: (1) women who begin to menstruate at a young age (9 to 10 years old), (2) women who reach menopause at an older age than average (54 to 55 years), (3) women who have never had children, (4) women who have their first baby after age 30, (5) women who menstruate for 40 or more years without a break (no pregnancy and no use of oral contraceptives), and (6) women who have been exposed to high levels of radiation (especially if exposure was during the time between the first period and the first pregnancy). Studies have shown breasts to be particularly susceptible to environmental carcinogens during the time between the first period and the first pregnancy.

In addition, there are certain pockets of the United States where the incidence of breast cancer is especially high. The Long Island Sound area of New York and Connecticut has an especially high number of breast cancer cases.

At one time it was speculated that breast-feeding had a protective effect, but this has been shown to be untrue in reliable studies. However, research indicates that women who have had their ovaries removed are at a decreased risk of developing breast cancer.

Symptoms

The most common symptom is a painless, irregular, firm lump in the breast. If this lump goes undetected during a breast self-exam or mammography, it will progress to create a dimpling in the skin or a retraction of the nipple. With the spread of the disease, swelling of the skin results in an enlargement of the skin pores. This will make the skin of the breast look something like an orange peel (referred to as peau d'orange). At this stage the cancer is very far advanced indeed, and the prognosis is extremely poor. Breast cancer commonly metastasizes (spreads) to the bones, liver, and brain, but other organs may also be involved.

Screening

The breast self-exam. There are currently three screening methods for breast cancer. The first is a breast self-exam, which is easy to teach, easy to do, and free. Most cancers of the breast are found this way, either by the woman herself or by her sexual partner. This technique should be learned and implemented at a young age, because the more familiar you are with the way your breasts normally feel, the sooner you will recognize when something is not right. What are you looking for? You are looking for something that is different.

Breasts consist of fatty tissue containing many milk (mammary) glands. Before your menstrual period (usually three to four days before), the glands in the breast swell up and become tender. They will feel lumpy when you touch them. After your period is over, the swelling in the glands goes down, making the breast self-exam more comfortable and easier to perform. Many women mistake swollen glands for a lump in their breast, so the timing of the exam is important.

One week after your period is generally a good time for the self-exam. The shower is the best place to do it—for three reasons: You are already undressed; wet, soapy skin allows your hand to slide over the breast more easily; and many women feel the shower is an acceptable place to feel their bodies, so they're more comfortable examining their breasts there.

The American Cancer Society as well as some pharmaceutical companies have printed up plastic-covered reminder cards for the self-exam, and they are made to fit over the shower head. The biggest drawback to the self-exam is that many women will not do it—even those who understand and acknowledge that it is valuable and important. The procedure for performing a breast self-exam is really quite simple. Some women have been misled and taught that it is a lengthy, complex procedure. It is not. The breast self-exam should not be intimidating. Feeling your breasts should be like feeling any other part of your body. Women never worry if their knuckles are normal or not; they get used to the normal lumps and learn to appreciate those lumps that are not normal.

You should start the exam by looking at your breasts in the mirror. Check to see that the nipple of each breast is similar in shape and location to that of the other breast. Breast masses can pull the nipple in, so this is an important observation. Check to see if there is any dimpling in the skin or change in contour from the previous month. These changes may also indicate that there is a breast mass.

Once in the shower, raise one arm up over your head. This flattens out the breast as much as possible. With the opposite hand, feel around the perimeter of your breast. When you have completed the circle, move your hand in from the circle toward the nipple. Once you reach the nipple, go back to the outer circle again, move your hand a little around the circle, and move it in toward the nipple again as if you were tracing bicycle spokes.

That is one way to do it, but there are others. The key is to cover the entire breast area without missing any spots. You may use concentric circles or vertical stripes; it really doesn't matter which pattern you use. Pick one that is comfortable for you and do it regularly. Any of these methods will allow you to feel the entire breast in a minute or less.

When you finish with one breast, repeat the exam of the other breast, again raising that arm up over your head. When you have finished, gently squeeze your nipples a little bit to check for any dis-

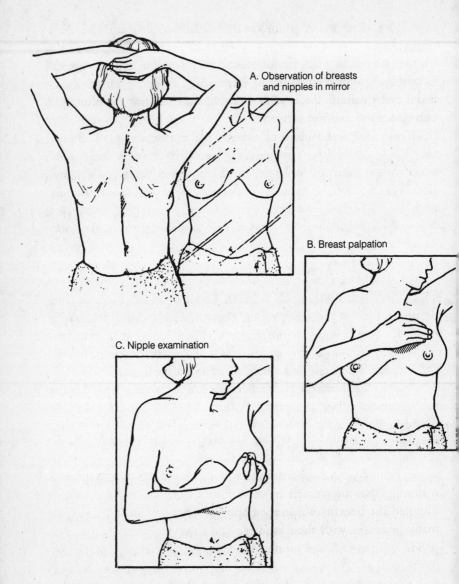

A. Observation of breasts and nipples in mirror

B. Breast palpation

C. Nipple examination

Figure 13.1. Breast Self-examination

charge. If you do feel something and you are not sure what it is, check the other breast in the same spot. If you feel the same thing there, it is usually nothing to worry about. Breast cancer occurs most commonly in one breast only, is irregular in shape, does not move around freely, and is rarely painful. If it is painful, it usually means that the lump is an enlarged gland and not cancer.

If you ever feel a lump or other tissue mass that you are unsure about, it is always a good idea to have your health-care provider check it out. If you can psychologically stand the wait, make the appointment for just after your next period, when the glands will be least engorged. It is not something you need to rush to the emergency room for; an appointment can be made for the earliest convenient time.

Mammography. Mammography is an excellent screening test for breast cancer, but there are some controversies associated with it. Many international studies done prior to the 1990s have shown a reduction in the death rates from breast cancer when mammography was used to screen women for early detection. It was those studies that led the American Cancer Society to issue its recommendation of (1) one baseline mammogram for women at age 40; (2) a mammogram every two years for women between the ages of 40 and 49, assuming the baseline was normal; and (3) yearly mammograms for women after age 50. It's been recommended that women with a strong family history of the disease have a yearly mammogram after age 40.

Recent studies have called into question the lifesaving benefit of mammography in women in their forties, whereas no studies have disputed the benefit of mammography in women over 50. There are many problems with these studies. The most important is that they divide women into age groups rather than into pre- and postmenopausal groups. The premenopausal breast is more difficult to image and, therefore, it is technically difficult to discern early breast masses. The postmenopausal breast has fewer prominent ducts and glands and is technically easier to image. In postmenopausal women, yearly mammograms are clearly documented to detect breast cancers before such cancers can be felt on examination. The survival rate for women whose breast cancers have been detected early is much greater than for those women who have later-stage tumors.

Most women have heard stories of how painful and humiliating it is to have a mammogram. The actual procedure should be neither. It is true that women with very small breasts may feel some pinching, but if the mammogram is done a week after your period, when there is little glandular swelling, the test may be uncomfortable, but should not be painful. Nor should it be embarrassing. The technicians who perform the mammogram are usually women, some of whom have been through the test themselves.

The procedure starts with a brief medical history and then a very low-dose X ray of each breast. The test is performed with you in the standing position, and two views of each breast are done. If there is a suspicious lump found by self-exam or by examination by your caregiver, that area is marked with a patch. The breast is stretched and compressed to be as flat as possible between glass plates, which are held at breast level. Your breast becomes the center of a "sandwich" between two plates. The actual picture taking lasts only a few seconds, and then your breast is released. The same procedure is done for the other breast. Some mammography clinics and units will give you the results right away; others will give the results to your caregiver, who in turn will notify you of the results.

Possible Risks   One reason that mammography is controversial is that about 5 percent of the women screened produce suspicious results. Of this small number, only 10 percent will have cancer. Therefore, it is argued that many unnecessary biopsies (procedures in which lumps are surgically removed and examined by a pathologist) are being performed.

There is also a question of the radiation exposure and possible risks from that. Yes, there is some exposure to radiation with mammography, but it should be compared realistically to everyday exposure. The dosage of radiation has been reduced drastically since mammography was first employed. The amount of radiation you receive now is approximately one-third of what you receive with a complete set of dental X rays. There are risks involved in everything we do.

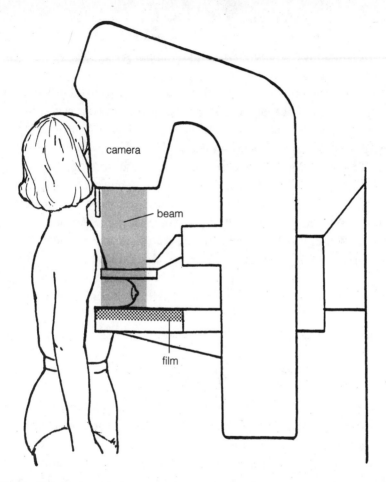

Figure 13.2. Mammography

They must be compared with the benefits, and the fact is that early detection of breast cancer leads to a better quality of life.

Ultrasound. In women under age 35, mammography as a screening test (i.e., if your breasts feel normal) is felt to be ineffective. Young women commonly have very dense breasts, which make the false-negative rate in mammography significantly high enough to render the test inconclusive. This means that mammography may not pick up breast cancer, even though it is present. If you feel a lump, however, mammography may be an important diagnostic tool.

If you do feel a lump, ultrasound can be used to differentiate solid lumps from fluid-filled lumps (cysts). However, it cannot detect microcalcifications, which are often the earliest signs of breast cancer. Ultrasound does not involve radiation; it uses sound waves to produce a picture. An ultrasound transducer is placed on the breast, and an image is shown on a screen similar to that of a television set.

The test is done while the woman is lying down with her arm up over her head. This flattens out the breast as much as possible. The technician puts some water-based jelly over the breast and applies the transducer, which he or she then moves around the entire area, watching the screen the whole time. As the transducer moves, the image on the screen moves and the technician can check different angles to get a more accurate idea of what is inside the breast. If something suspicious appears on the screen, the technician freezes the image and takes a picture of it. Ultrasound takes more time to perform than mammography, which takes only a few minutes.

Treatment

The treatment of breast cancer varies widely and should be individualized to the woman herself. The only real treatment advances have been in early detection. Otherwise, surgery is almost always involved in some way. The options include a partial mastectomy, a lumpectomy with radiation therapy, or a modified radical mastectomy. The decision about the type of treatment is based on many factors: the woman's family history, age, menopausal status, size of the tumor, size of the breast, access to properly administered radiation care, and the woman's feelings about what she is willing to accept.

Current medical treatment for breast cancer is extremely invasive and life-altering. At present, there are no alternative therapies that have any curative effects. Surgery, chemotherapy, and radiation all have major side effects that cause a great deal of pain and discomfort. Yet for many women, those treatments cause temporary discomfort and are the trade-offs that prolong life. Treatment for breast cancer, however unpleasant, can lead to many happy and disease-free years.

If mastectomy is an appropriate treatment and has been chosen by you, your partner, and your physician, breast reconstruction surgery can be performed at the time of your mastectomy or at a later date. This is an appropriate option for some women, although there are some risks involved.

Breast reconstruction is a procedure in which an artificial breast is created by a plastic surgeon, using either silicone or saline implants or tissue taken from elsewhere in the body. The new breast will give you a natural contour, especially under clothing, but you will have no sexual feeling in it. This surgery helps many women feel more "normal" and helps greatly to resolve a certain sense of loss for them. Breast reconstruction, however, carries an additional risk of infection, and the long-term effects of artificial implants are controversial and unknown. For this reason, it is not an option for every woman.

After a mastectomy, many women wear a breast prosthesis that has been custom-made to match the remaining breast. This is a breast-shaped device that fits into a bra, so when you are clothed, the loss of a breast is not noticeable. The American Cancer Society is a wonderful resource for breast prostheses, and the Society sends breast cancer survivors to visit women before they leave the hospital. These individuals are trained to counsel other women about breast prostheses as well as about other aspects of living with this disease.

Sex After Breast Cancer

Resuming sexual activity after breast cancer treatment is completely dependent on how you and your partner feel. The loss of one or both breasts can be devastating to a woman's self-image. Breasts are a symbol of femininity and sexuality, and mastectomy is an amputative procedure. It may take many months of grieving before you are able to enjoy sex again. Professional counseling is always a good idea to help cope with the loss, and support groups are especially helpful.

Radiation and chemotherapy can make you feel quite terrible physically. It is difficult to enjoy any kind of sexual experience when feeling nauseated, fatigued, and frightened, so give yourself some time. An understanding and compassionate partner is the greatest gift a woman can have after enduring such a loss. To feel wanted and attractive is always a comfort and relief. Ideally, a couple should get counseling together, as sexual partners must also go through the grieving process. Be as open about your feelings as possible. Crying is normal and should not be repressed. As always, open communication and mutual respect for each other's feelings is the optimal way to make it through a very difficult time.

If your breasts were a major part of your sexual activity, the actual physical act of foreplay or sexual intercourse will obviously have to change to some degree. Some women find that if their remaining breast is fondled during sex, all their anxieties surrounding the disease suddenly well up. Experiment with different techniques and settings. You may be more comfortable in the dark for a while until you are more accustomed to the way your body looks. It also may be helpful for you to wear a breast prosthesis under some attractive nightgowns. There are women, however, who find shopping for negligees to be very depressing and upsetting after recent surgery. See how you feel about it. When you are ready, experiment with your partner. Changing your sexual routine often helps to keep the excitement going.

Prevention

Unfortunately, breast cancer is not a preventable disease. Until much more effort and money are put into researching causes for breast cancer, its control is completely dependent on early detection and proper treatment.

CERVICAL CANCER

Cancer of the uterine cervix is nearly 100 percent curable. It is the most easily detectable and treatable form of cancer in women.

Incidence

At the present time there is no reason why any woman should die of cervical cancer, but many do. In the United States alone, about 7,400 deaths occur annually from cervical cancer. The incidence is increased in women of lower socioeconomic status, and in those who have a history of sexually transmitted diseases.

Risk Factors

Unlike breast cancer, there are some specific factors that will put you at an increased risk of getting cervical cancer. The first one is starting sexual activity at an early age (adolescence). Multiple sexual partners will also increase your risk, and if you have many sexual partners starting early in your teens, the risk is increased even more. Cervical cancer is more common in cigarette smokers. Recent studies have shown that barrier methods of contraception (condoms, diaphragms, cervical caps) reduce the risk of cervical cancer. Women who have never had sexual intercourse will rarely develop cervical cancer.

Women whose mothers took diethylstilbestrol (DES) while pregnant during the 1950s or 1960s have an increased risk of cervical cell changes. These changes rarely lead to cervical cancer, but they may.

Symptoms

The symptoms of cervical cancer are slight or nonexistent. Occasionally, there may be a thin, watery, or bloody discharge. In rare instances, women might experience some bleeding after intercourse. If the disease is advanced, more episodes of bleeding between periods or after menopause may be noted. In addition, more advanced cervical cancer is often accompanied by pelvic pain.

Screening

The reason that invasive cervical cancer is so effectively treatable is the availability of one simple and effective screening test: the Pap smear. If every woman had a Pap smear on a regular basis, deaths from cervical cancer would be extremely rare. The National Institutes of Health offer these guidelines: (1) All young women should have an initial Pap smear at the onset of sexual activity; (2) even if the initial Pap smear is negative, yearly Pap smears should be performed; and (3) women who have never had sexual intercourse need not have regular Pap smears unless they were exposed to DES in utero.

The Pap smear is a very reliable test for cervical cell changes leading to cancer. If the smear shows abnormal changes, the woman must then go through a more definitive diagnostic procedure called colposcopy. The colposcope is basically a pair of binoculars set on a base with a very good light source. It is positioned a few inches from the vaginal opening, and a speculum is put in place to expose the cervix. The cervix is then washed with several applications of a mild vinegar solution. With the cervix brightly lit and magnified, any surfaces that might harbor abnormal cells will appear different from those with normal cervical cells. Tiny pieces of this cervical tissue are removed (biopsied) and sent to a pathologist for analysis. The extent of the abnormality is graded by the pathologist as mild, moderate, or severe dysplasia (cervical cell changes) or actual cervical cancer. Dysplasia can be treated very easily before the cells become cancerous.

Colposcopy may be performed as an office procedure by a physician, nurse-practitioner, or physician's assistant. If your health-care provider has not been trained in colposcopy, you will be referred to his or her consulting physician for this diagnostic test. A woman may receive the results of her test by contacting the practitioner who performed the exam, not the lab or lab pathologist.

Treatment

The treatment for cervical cancer depends on the stage of the disease. Very early findings may be treated on an outpatient basis with cryotherapy (freezing) of the cervix, laser, or surgical removal of the lesion. Invasive cancer that has spread into the cervix or to other organs will require hospitalization, a hysterectomy, and/or radiation treatments in consultation with a gynecologic oncologist.

Prevention

If one studies the risk factors for cervical cancer, it would follow that delaying sexual intercourse is an obvious preventive action. Very young women should be told that intercourse at a young age puts them at risk not only for pregnancy and sexually transmitted diseases but also for cervical cancer. If a woman in her adolescent years decides that she wants to become sexually active, she should protect herself from these conditions by the regular use of condoms. Women should also limit the number of sexual partners they have in order to reduce their risk of cervical cancer, sexually transmitted diseases, and AIDS.

OVARIAN CANCER

Incidence

The incidence of ovarian cancer, like many other types of cancer, is steadily increasing. The ovaries are unique, since they consist of a variety of tissue types and are therefore susceptible to different types of cancers. Very young women in their teens and early twenties more commonly develop cancers derived from the germ cell layers of the ovaries. These types of cancers have a better prognosis and rate of cure after surgical removal and aggressive chemotherapy than the cancers typically found in older women.

Women who are perimenopausal and older tend to experience cancers that affect the outer layer of the ovary. Approximately 80 percent of all ovarian cancers are of this type. They are found almost exclusively in white women and are most common in those who never had children, have never been on the birth control pill, or are of Jewish heritage. There are other types of ovarian cancers that affect both white and black women, but these are less widespread. In general, ovarian cancer has a poor survival rate. This is due in part to the advanced stage of the disease when it is diagnosed. Ovarian cancer, unlike breast cancer, grows and spreads very quickly, with few if any warning signs or symptoms.

Risk Factors

High-risk groups for ovarian cancer have not been clearly identified. However, several studies have shown some tendencies that may be possible risk factors. The disease is more prevalent in women who have had little or no interruption in ovulation (such as women who have never given birth), who started their menses very early, or who have not been on oral contraceptive pills. Other studies have shown that infertility and early menopause can increase one's risk. Environmental factors such as pelvic irradiation and exposure to talc and asbestos have also been mentioned as possible risk factors, but with little substantiation. Ovarian cancer is more common in women of higher socioeconomic classes and/or who have relatives with breast or ovarian cancer.

Symptoms

The earliest symptoms of ovarian cancer are usually quite vague and nonspecific. Pain during intercourse may sometimes be an early symptom of ovarian cancer. Gastrointestinal symptoms, which are the most common initial complaints, include bloating, excessive gas, and loss of appetite. Some women with ovarian cancer will notice an unexplained weight loss accompanied by an expanding waistline. A very distended abdomen or a mass that can be felt in the abdomen indicates that the disease is very advanced.

Screening

Ovarian cancer is usually found on a routine gynecological exam. After the speculum exam, your health-care practitioner will perform a bimanual exam (described in chapter 3). During this exam, he or she places one hand on your abdomen and one or two fingers inside your vagina. In this way, it is possible to feel the size and shape of your reproductive organs, including the ovaries. If the ovaries seem larger than normal size or have an abnormal shape, you will then be referred for diagnostic tests that include pelvic ultrasound and blood tests. These are currently the only ways to detect ovarian cancer.

Ultrasound is a noninvasive test that produces a picture of your internal organs using sound waves. The ovaries are best visualized by vaginal ultrasound, a test done with the transducer of the ultrasound placed in the vagina. This picture is transmitted to a screen and can be evaluated by a specialist, usually a radiologist.

Ultrasound can distinguish between ovarian cysts and solid ovarian masses. A cyst is much more common in ovulating women and is not associated with cancer or long-term illness. Any ovarian mass felt on exam should be evaluated by ultrasound, especially in prepubescent girls and menopausal women. The chances of finding a cyst in those groups are less likely but require expedient diagnosis and treatment.

Although routine gynecological exams are extremely important in determining normal pelvic anatomy, they usually do not pick up early ovarian cancers because they cause ovarian enlargement only in the later stages of the disease.

For women with a strong family history of ovarian cancer (mother, sister, or daughter), a screening protocol had been proposed. This involved a pelvic exam combined with a vaginal ultrasound of the ovaries. These examinations were performed every six months. Three months after each pelvic exam and ultrasound, a blood test for the ovarian tumor marker CA-125 was taken. This means that every three months some evaluation of the ovaries was done. Unfortunately, recent studies have shown this protocol to be ineffective in early diagnosis and alteration of the course of ovarian cancer.

The CA-125 blood test has been touted by many as an ovarian cancer screening test for all women, but that assessment is inaccurate. This test in no way guarantees detection of ovarian cancer in its earliest stages, and actually might offer a false sense of security to those at highest risk. In addition, there are many false-positive findings, which may result in unnecessary surgery for a nonexistent tumor.

Treatment

The treatment of ovarian cancer involves surgery, which can be extensive. The uterus, fallopian tubes, and ovaries are usually removed, along with any other affected areas. A woman faced with this type of surgery should have ample time to discuss the procedure with the surgeon, and *all* of her questions should be thoroughly answered. It is recommended that the surgery be performed as quickly as possible because of the rapid spread of this type of cancer. After surgery, most patients undergo some form of chemotherapy, usually for a period of six months, and some may continue treatment for up to a full year. Follow-up treatment may require further surgery and/or radiation. Because most cases of ovarian cancer are discovered in advanced stages of the disease, five-year survival rates are very low.

Prevention

Currently there are no proven methods of preventing ovarian cancer. Those with a strong family history bear close scrutiny. A few aggressive gynecologists actually recommend prophylactic removal of the ovaries in high-risk women, although even this radical treatment may not prevent the development of the disease.

UTERINE CANCER

Incidence

Cancer of the uterus affects more women in the United States than does either cervical cancer or ovarian cancer. Approximately 45,000 new cases are diagnosed in this country every year, and the disease most commonly affects menopausal women between age 51 and 60. Only about 5 percent of all cases are diagnosed before age 40.

Risk Factors

The women who are at higher risk for uterine cancer are obese women, women who have never given birth, and women who are exposed to estrogen without progesterone. Estrogen, when used alone, is associated with a three- to sevenfold increase in the risk of cancer of the endometrium, the lining of the uterus. This may be caused by estrogen taken by mouth or produced in excessive amounts within the body. These internal sources include estrogen-secreting tumors as well as the high levels of estrogen found in extremely obese women. (Such women have a constantly elevated supply of estrogen because fat cells produce estrogen.) Estrogen replacement therapy should not be given to women who still have a uterus unless the estrogen is complemented by progesterone therapy.

Hormone supplements during and after menopause that employ a cyclic or simultaneous dosage of estrogen and progesterone seem to protect the uterine lining from developing cancer. Women with family histories of uterine cancer are at a higher risk of getting the disease, and those who have a history of breast, ovarian, or colon cancer also have a greater risk of developing uterine cancer.

Symptoms

Usually, the first symptom of cancer of the uterus is postmenopausal vaginal bleeding. Women who are going through menopause will often manifest irregular, heavy, frequent, or prolonged periods. Those symptoms can occur as normal occurrences or as a symptom of the disease. In premenopausal women, the symptoms may also include spotting between periods or after intercourse, and frequent, irregular, or heavy periods. Since the symptoms may not differ in perimenopausal women, a biopsy should be performed. All postmenopausal bleeding must be investigated to rule out cancer.

Screening

At present the only screening test for diagnosis of uterine cancer is an endometrial biopsy, hysteroscopy with biopsy, or D&C. The endometrial biopsy (removal and analysis of endometrial tissue) can be done on an outpatient basis in an office setting. A biopsy is more invasive than a Pap smear, and many women find it extremely uncomfortable. It involves inserting an instrument (a small curette) through the cervix into the uterus, where cells are obtained by scraping the inner walls of the uterine lining. Some argue that the biopsy is not a conclusive test because the biopsied area may not represent the entire endometrium, and some cancers may be missed. Nevertheless, such an oversight would be very unusual, since the office biopsy will take cells from the front, back, and sides of the uterine lining.

The hysteroscopy, which can be performed with or without general anesthesia, involves inserting a thin, periscope-like instrument through the cervix into the uterus. The uterine lining can then be visualized, and cell samples from abnormal areas can be obtained with a biopsy instrument.

A D&C, which is usually performed under general anesthesia, involves dilating the cervical opening to accommodate a curette, a sharp, spoon-shaped instrument designed to scrape off the cells of the uterine lining.

Ultrasound may be used to visualize the uterine lining. If the lining is not thickened, then endometrial cancer is unlikely. However, ultrasound does not get a picture of the cell type inside the uterus and is therefore not a definitive test for endometrial cancer.

Treatment

The treatment for uterine cancer depends on the stage of the disease when it is diagnosed. A hysterectomy is usually indicated, with radiation therapy before or after the hysterectomy. The stage of the disease usually determines whether the radiation is given before or after the hysterectomy (or both). More advanced uterine cancers may also require chemotherapy, although this is rare.

Prevention

A healthful diet and avoidance of obesity will help in preventing uterine cancer; however, it is not a guarantee. Unopposed estrogen will substantially increase the risk of uterine cancer, and this should be clearly understood if you are considering hormone replacement therapy (see chapter 11). Prompt treatment of any abnormal pelvic mass (a possible estrogen-producing tumor) will also reduce the risk of uterine cancer. Any woman who has irregular or abnormal bleeding, particularly during or after menopause, must have an evaluation of the uterine lining performed. This may be done by office biopsy, hysteroscopy with biopsy, or with dilation and curettage.

14

GUARDING AGAINST INAPPROPRIATE CARE

The most important thing you can do to protect yourself from inappropriate care is to be well informed. Knowing your body and how it works is the cornerstone of good health. Preventive care—including regular exercise, a healthful diet, and appropriate cancer screening (Pap smear, mammography)—should be an integral part of your life. Avoiding unhealthful habits (smoking, drug or alcohol abuse) will improve your chances for a long life. Sexual health is an out-growth of both a healthful lifestyle and an understanding of (and pride in) your body.

There are safeguards in the American medical system to prevent inappropriate treatments, but certain practitioners find many ways to get around the system if they are determined to do so. Any health-care provider can misuse his or her position. Medical procedures such as colposcopies and surgical procedures such as hysterectomies must be performed only by people who are trained and certified care providers.

You should always feel comfortable with your health-care provider and the treatment the two of you have agreed upon. *The treatment must suit the diagnosis.* If you are at all uncomfortable with the treatment suggested, you should not hesitate to get a second opinion. If the practitioner you are seeing won't allow a second opinion, leave him or her immediately and find another caregiver.

How to choose a caregiver is discussed in chapter 2. You should know something about the person you are choosing as a care provider. Find out if he or she is someone who keeps moving from place to place, and if so, why. If the caregiver has any requests, demands, or practices you feel are aberrant or unreasonable, find someone else to care for you.

If you are having sexual problems, you may be particularly at risk for succumbing to unreasonable or aberrant practices. Most women in our culture find it difficult to discuss sexual issues or, for that matter, any issues involving the genitals. Many people don't even know the proper anatomical terms (e.g., "I'm having a problem 'down there' "). Many are embarrassed to bring up sexual issues with their regular caregivers, so they may seek people they don't really know and who won't know them, their family, or friends. The key to avoiding unreasonable treatments in the field of women's sexual health is to overcome your embarrassment, learn more about your body and how it works, and be proud of it. If women could get over the shame of their life cycles, periods, pregnancies, and menopause, they would be less vulnerable to unnecessary treatments and procedures.

Alternative therapies such as acupuncture, chiropractic, herbology, yoga, spiritual healing, and massage therapy are not unreasonable treatments. Even though they are not based on Western scientific practice, they have a traditional or spiritual basis that many people find helpful. Not every mode of treatment is appropriate for every person. Many people see chemotherapy as poison, yet the medical world sees it as an appropriate treatment for cancer. Chemotherapy certainly has a place in the treatment of cancer, but it can be given with some forms of alternative therapy.

You should never feel railroaded into a treatment, especially if you have reviewed and investigated it but have still decided against it. Patients (especially women) who are in pain or have a serious disease are vulnerable. They may be coerced into therapies with which they are not totally comfortable. It is for this reason that every woman, before she has a serious illness, should have a health-care provider whom she trusts and with whom she is at ease. Even with such a care provider, you should be seeking answers and explanations. Nothing should ever happen to your body without your understanding why. You should also be aware of what alternatives there may be. The days of having surgery "because my doctor told me I had to" should be gone forever. You should take just as big a part in the decision-making process as your health-care provider does. You must understand that you alone have the power to make the ultimate decisions regarding your health and well-being. You deserve good health care.

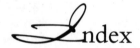

Index